6 WEEKS
TO
SUPERHEALTH

Other books by Patrick Holford

Optimum Nutrition Bible
100% Health
The 30-Day Fatburner Diet
Beat Stress and Fatigue
Say No To Cancer
Say No To Heart Disease
Say No To Arthritis
Improve Your Digestion
Balancing Hormones Naturally (with Kate Neil)
Boost Your Immune System (with Jennifer Meek)
Supplements for Superhealth
The Optimum Nutrition Cookbook (with Judy Ridgway)
Mental Health and Illness – The Nutrition Connection (ION Press)

6 WEEKS TO SUPER HEALTH

AN EASY-TO-FOLLOW PROGRAMME FOR TOTAL HEALTH TRANSFORMATION

PATRICK HOLFORD

PIATKUS

First published in 2000 by
Judy Piatkus (Publishers) Ltd
5 Windmill Street, London W1P 1HF
E-mail: info@piatkus.co.uk

For the latest news and information on all our titles
visit our new website at www.piatkus.co.uk

The moral rights of the author have been asserted

A catalogue record for this book is available from the British Library

ISBN 0-7499-1963-9

Designed by Paul Saunders
Typeset by Phoenix Photosetting, Chatham, Kent
Printed and bound in Great Britain by
Butler & Tanner Ltd, Frome, Somerset

Contents

Acknowledgements

This book would not have been possible without the help and support of many people. I am indebted to Oscar Ichazo for his generous permission to include the exercise programme from *Master Level Exercise Psychocalisthenics*, and to Judy Ridgway for her generous permission to include recipes from *The Optimum Nutrition Cookbook*. A very special thanks goes to Natalie Savona and Sharon Kaye who worked with me to create the 6-week strategy, and to Bebe Kohlap for taking care of things in my absence. Last but not least to Rachel Winning and her team for their painstaking editing and design.

Psychocalisthenics is a registered trademark of Arica Institute, Inc.

Guide to Abbreviations and Measures

1 pound (lb) = 16 ounces (oz)   2.2lb = 1 kilogram (kg)
1 pint = 0.6 litres   1.76 pints = 1 litre
2 teaspoons (tsp) = 1 dessertspoon (dsp)
1.5 dessertspoons = 1 tablespoon (tbsp)
In this book, calories means kilocalories (kcal)

PART 1

DEFINING SUPERHEALTH

Feeling Just 'All Right' Isn't All Right

6 Steps to Superhealth

How Healthy Are You?

Feeling Just 'All Right' Isn't All Right

Health isn't just an absence of illness, it's the abundance of vitality. I believe there exists for all of us the tangible and achievable experience of a profound sense of well-being. This is characterised by a consistent, clear and high level of energy, an emotional balance, a sharp mind, a desire to maintain physical fitness and a direct awareness of what suits our bodies, what enhances our health, and what our needs are in any given moment. This state of health includes a resilience to infectious diseases and protection from the major killer diseases such as heart disease and cancer; it consequently means slowing down the ageing process and living a long and healthy life. At its most profound level health is not merely the absence of pain or tension, but a joy in living, a real appreciation of what it is to have a healthy body with which to taste the many pleasures of this world.

For me, this is not just a belief but an experience which I have myself and which I have witnessed in so many other people with whom I have worked over the past 17 years since I started to pursue 'optimum nutrition'. Health has not been a static state, but an endless journey of learning about myself from the diseases and imbalances that I have suffered, and a continuing discovery of even higher and clearer levels of energy.

Check Your Health Balance

Imagine that you are born with a health reserve – a certain amount of money in your health deposit account. Depending what you eat, drink, breathe and think, gradually money is lost from that health deposit account. Once you go overdrawn your energy is low, you can't get out of bed in the morning and you suffer from niggling health problems, from colds to PMS. As your overdraft grows you develop diseases and when you exceed your overdraft limit that's when you die! Of course, it's only at the disease stage that conventional medicine kicks in. Once you are horizontally ill, their job is to get you vertical again – functioning but not necessarily superhealthy. Most people are walking around vertically ill – standing up but hardly bounding about full of the joys of spring.

SUPERHEALTH	VERTICALLY ILL	HORIZONTALLY ILL
boundless energy	constant tiredness	chronic fatigue
perspective on life	drained	exhausted
sharp mind	low concentration	constant aches
positive outlook	mood swings	depression
joie de vivre	exhausted by exercise	pessimism
physically fit	unfit	unable to exercise
rarely/never ill	run down and frequently ill	incapacitated by illness
full life	easily overwhelmed	life is hard work
toned body	flabby	life is against me
contentment	dissatisfaction	despair

How is your health account?

Take a look at the columns above. Where are you? A great number of people fall into the Vertically Ill category – lacking enthusiasm for life. How would it be to sit comfortably and consistently in the superhealth category – full of energy in both mind and body? This is what we are aiming for in this book, and not just during the 6 Weeks to Superhealth programme but for you to take with you for the rest of your life.

While many of my other books help you prevent and reverse diseases (*Say No to Heart Disease, Say No to Cancer, Say No to Arthritis* – see the full list on page 218), this book is a highly practical 6-week strategy to regain superhealth. The science of superhealth is all about building up your health reserve so that not only do you not get sick but you also experience superhealth, with plenty of capacity to adapt to stressful times.

Instead of measuring whether or not you have a disease, the science of superhealth starts by measuring how well you are functioning – whether you are firing on all cylinders. The objective is to improve your health status before chronic disease develops. This approach is known as 'functional medicine' and focuses on the early detection and correction of imbalances as a means to understand, prevent and reverse disease.

The Four Aspects of Superhealth

There's a Zen Buddhist saying that 'Health isn't everything. But without health everything is nothing.' While there is truth to the saying that you are what you eat, we are more than that. We are physical, chemical and psychological beings and we live in an environment. An imbalance in any one of these domains can deplete your health. The four aspects of superhealth are:

1. **Optimum nutrition,** which seeks to perfect the balance of the body on a chemical level.

2. **Fitness,** which seeks to perfect the balance on a physical level.

3. **The right attitude,** which seeks to perfect the balance on a mental and emotional level.

4. **A healthy environment,** which seeks to perfect the environment in which we live.

Then there is the spiritual dimension, which we can define as our 'connectedness' with others, our environment and ourselves. In Oriental systems this also relates to 'chi' or 'prana', vital energy that we can tap into when our mind and

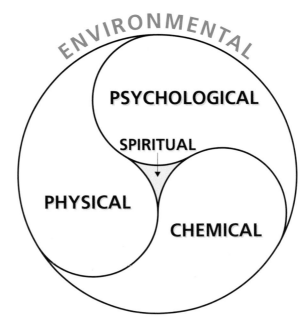

The Four Aspects of Superhealth

body are in harmony. Yoga and tai chi, for example, are forms of exercise specifically designed to generate vital energy by bringing the mind and body into harmony. This vital energy comes to us through food and through breathing and can also be generated internally by being in the right state of mind.

The fastest way to attain superhealth is to tune yourself up on every level. In each of the 6 Weeks to Superhealth you'll find:

- **A dietary strategy** packed with high-vitality foods and excluding foods, drinks and patterns of eating that deplete energy.

- **Specific supplements** to improve your digestion, cleanse your body, boost your immune system, generate mental and physical energy and balance your hormones.

- **Awareness exercises** that will generate mental clarity and emotional balance, and bring you into a more conscious relationship with your body, with food and your immediate environment.

- **A unique exercise system** that incorporates specific breathing patterns with physical exercises, designed to generate vitality and bring your mind and body into harmony.

Each of these vital aspects of your 6 Weeks to Superhealth is explained in Part 2. Make sure you read this section of the book and understand the basic principles before starting the 6-week strategy detailed in Part 3. Each week has a specific focus, based on 6 fundamental body processes – the 6 steps to health.

6 Steps to Superhealth

There are 6 key steps, or processes in the body, that reflect where you are on the scale from disease to superhealth. Almost all diseases result from an imbalance in one or more of these 6 key processes. On the other hand, if you're firing at 100 per cent on all cylinders you are superhealthy and very unlikely to get sick. The purpose of 6 Weeks to Superhealth is to tune up each of the fundamental processes shown below.

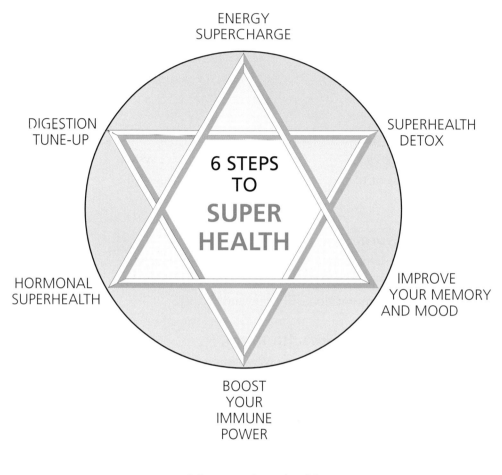

6 Steps to Superhealth

In addition you will have learned an entire exercise routine called *Psychocalisthenics*, and developed a much greater awareness and improved relationship with your body, with food and with your health. You will have regained control of your own vitality and, in short, will know what to do to live a long, healthy and rewarding life.

Since we are all different, some weeks will be more important for you than others. These, understandably, may be harder and will require more effort on your part. Having seen in thousands of people the extraordinary results that can be achieved in a very short time by following these guidelines, I urge you to put 100 per cent into following the indications for each of the 6 weeks. The more thoroughly you follow each week the more you will experience an improvement in your health.

- ## Week 1 – Energy Supercharge

The first week gives you an energy supercharge by improving your ability to keep your blood sugar level even. This is critical for energy, but also for stress resistance and weight control. By the end of Week 1 you should experience a new level of energy and take life in your stride.

- ## Week 2 – Digestion Tune-up

The second week cleans up and tunes up your digestive system so you can really get the most out of the healthy foods you are eating, as well as improving your elimination.

- ## Week 3 – Hormonal Superhealth

Whether you are a man or a woman and whatever your stage in the life cycle, the third week helps you balance your hormones, which have effects on your emotional balance, motivation, sex drive and vitality.

- ## Week 4 – The Superhealth Detox

By the fourth week you will be ready for the superhealth detox – a chance to really spring-clean your system and restore your liver's ability to detoxify the many harmful substances the body creates every day, as well as those we take in from impure food, air and water.

- ## Week 5 – Boost Your Immune Power

Having eliminated many of the foods and drinks that are most likely to cause allergies, here's your chance in the fifth week to find out which foods you're particularly sensitive to and which foods you can safely bring back into your diet. In addition, you'll be learning how to improve your immune power and fight infections naturally.

- ## Week 6 – Improve Your Memory and Mood

In the final week you'll find out what to eat to improve your memory, concentration and mood. By this stage you will have learned how to prepare, cook and incorporate healthy foods into your life.

> To find out how healthy you are, and how healthy you could be, complete the **Superhealth Questionnaire** now.

How Healthy Are You?

The **Superhealth Questionnaire** is based on assessing each of the 6 steps to superhealth. Completing this questionnaire has two purposes. It gives you a measure of where you are now on a scale of health, and where you can be. At the end of the 6-week programme the questionnaire will be repeated so that you can reassess yourself and see how much progress you have made towards a higher level of health. The sections you score high on are also good pointers to the areas of your health that need the greatest attention.

SUPERHEALTH QUESTIONNAIRE

Score the questionnaire as follows:

0 for rarely or never
1 for sometimes
2 for frequently or always

Mark down your total for each of the 6 sections and your overall score.

1. Energy Check

- Are you still sleepy 20 minutes after getting up?
- Do you need tea, coffee, a cigarette or something to get you going in the morning?
- Do you crave sweet foods, bread, cereal, popcorn or pasta?
- Do you feel like you 'need' an alcoholic drink on most days?
- Are you overweight and unable to shift the extra pounds?
- Do you often have energy slumps during the day or after meals?
- Do you often have mood swings or difficulty concentrating?
- Do you get dizzy or irritable if you go 6 hours without food?
- Do you often find you over-react to stress?
- Is your energy now less than it used to be?

Section Total

2. Digestion Check

C　T

- Do you fail to chew your food thoroughly? ▢ 0 ◯
- Do you suffer from bad breath? ▢ 0 ◯
- Do you get a burning sensation in your stomach or regularly use indigestion tablets? ▢ 0 ◯
- Do you have a feeling of fullness in your stomach? ▢ 2 ◯
- Do you find it difficult digesting fatty foods? ▢ 0 ◯
- Do you get diarrhoea? ▢ 2 ◯
- Do you get constipation? ▢ 0 ◯
- Do you often get a bloated stomach or feel nauseous? ▢ 1 ◯
- Do you often belch or pass wind? ▢ 1　2
- Do you fail to have a bowel movement at least once a day? ▢ 0 ◯

Section Total ▢ 6　2

3. Hormone Check

Women

- Do you use the contraceptive pill? ▢ 2
- Do you often suffer from cyclical mood swings or depression? ▢ 0
- Do you experience cyclical water retention? ▢ 0
- Do you especially crave foods premenstrually? ▢ 0
- Have you at any time been bothered with problems affecting your reproductive organs (ovaries, womb)? ▢ 0
- Do you have fertility problems, difficulty conceiving or a history of miscarriage? ▢ 0
- Do you suffer from breast tenderness? ▢ 0
- Do you experience cramps or other menstrual irregularities? ▢ 0
- Are your periods often irregular or heavy? ▢ 0
- Do you suffer from reduced libido or loss of interest in sex? ▢ 0

Section Total ▢ 2

Men

T

- Have you had a vasectomy?
- Are you gaining weight?
- Do you often suffer from mood swings or depression?
- Have you at any time been bothered with problems affecting your reproductive organs (prostate or testes)?
- Do you suffer from reduced libido or loss of interest in sex?
- Do you suffer from impotence?
- Do you awake less frequently with a morning erection or have difficulty maintaining an erection?
- Do you suffer from fatigue or loss of energy?
- Have you had a drop in your motivation and drive?
- Do you feel that you are ageing prematurely?

Section Total 1

4. Detoxification Check

C   T

- Do you suffer from headaches or migraine?
- Do you have watery or itchy eyes or swollen, red or sticky eyelids or bags or dark circles under your eyes?
- Do you have itchy ears, earache, ear infections, drainage from the ears or ringing in the ears?
- Do you suffer from excessive mucus, a stuffy nose or sinus problems?
- Do you suffer from acne or skin rashes or hives?
- Do you sweat a lot and have a strong body odour?
- Do you have joint or muscle aches or pains?
- Do you have a sluggish metabolism and find it hard to lose weight, or are you underweight and find it hard to gain weight?
- Do you suffer from nausea or vomiting?
- Do you have a bitter taste in your mouth or a furry tongue?

Section Total 2   6

5. Immunity Check

C   T

- Do you get more than 3 colds a year?
- Do you get a stomach bug each year?
- Do you find it hard to shift an infection (cold or otherwise)?
- Are you prone to thrush or cystitis?
- Do you take at least one course of antibiotics each year?
- Is there any history of cancer in your family?
- Do the glands in your neck, armpits or groin feel tender?
- Do you suffer from allergy problems?
- Do you take any drugs or medicines?
- Do you have an inflammatory disease such as eczema, asthma or arthritis?

Section Total 2   2

6. Memory and Mood Check

C   T

- Is your memory deteriorating?
- Do you find it hard to concentrate and often get confused?
- Are you depressed?
- Do you become anxious easily or wake up with a feeling of anxiety?
- Does stress leave you feeling exhausted?
- Do you have mood swings and easily become angry or irritable?
- Are you lacking in motivation?
- Do you feel like you're 'out of control' of things?
- Do you have misperceptions where things don't look or sound right or you feel distant or disconnected?
- Do you suffer from insomnia?

Section Total 5   0

Overall Total 28   8

Your Score

- **If you score a total of 9 or more in any of the 6 sections**, these are the weeks to which you will have to give particular attention and follow the recommendations very carefully.

- **A score above 14 for any one section** indicates that this aspect of your health may well be struggling. It would be a good idea to keep following the guidelines for that specific week until your score is much lower and your health in that area is improved. By doing this you will have a tailored programme specifically designed for your individual needs.

- **If your total score is 60 or more**, it's definitely a great idea for you to be doing the 6 Weeks to Superhealth programme. It means your body is not doing such a great job of coping with your diet, lifestyle and/or environment, so you really do need to take a look at these as you work through your 6 weeks. It is especially important that you follow the recommendations given throughout, particularly during the weeks for which you scored highly.

- **If you scored between 30 and 60**, your health is at a stage where it could well do with the support of this 6-week programme to propel you towards superhealth. Remember to take particular care during the weeks where you scored 11 or more.

- **A total score of less than 30** means that you have a reasonable level of health reserve. 6 Weeks to Superhealth will help you jump to a higher level of health, with even more money in your health deposit account.

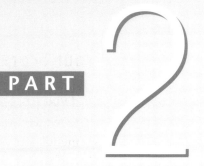

THE BASICS

BASIC PRINCIPLE 1

The Superhealth Diet

Before you embark on the 6 Weeks to Superhealth programme it is important to understand a few basic principles, the first of which is the Superhealth Diet. The basis of this diet is to provide an optimal intake of protein, fat, carbohydrate, vitamins, minerals and phytonutrients. While each week includes specific instructions to, for example, detoxify your body or balance your blood sugar or improve your digestion, the dietary recommendations are all based on providing an optimally balanced diet, based on my research at the Institute for Optimum Nutrition over the past 15 years. Our conclusions to date are shown in the Perfect Diet Pyramid. The general guidelines are as follows:

The Perfect Diet Pyramid

Fat
1 heaped tablespoon ground seeds or 1 tablespoon cold-pressed seed oil.

Protein
3 servings beans, lentils, quinoa, tofu (soya) or 'seed' vegetables. Occasionally replace one of these with a small helping of fish, cheese, a free-range egg or lean meat.

Complex Carbohydrates
4 servings of wholegrains, such as brown rice, millet, rye, oats, wholewheat, corn, quinoa, bread or pasta.

Fruit and Vegetables
6 servings of fruit and vegetables. Eat citrus fruits, apples, pears, berries and melons. The best vegetables are dark green, leafy and root vegetables.

Fat

There are two kinds of fat: saturated (hard) fat and unsaturated fat. It is neither essential to eat saturated fat, nor ideal to eat too much. Its main sources are meat and dairy products. Unsaturated fats can be further divided into two types: monounsaturated fats, found in olive oil; and polyunsaturated fats, found in nut and seed oils or in fish. Certain polyunsaturated fats are essential to the diet. These are called linoleic and linolenic acid and they are vital for the brain and nervous system, the immune system, the cardiovascular system and the skin. (A common sign of deficiency is dry skin.) The optimal diet provides a balance of these two essential fats, also known as Omega 3 and Omega 6 oils. Pumpkin and flax seeds are rich in linolenic acid (Omega 3), while sesame and sunflower seeds are rich in linoleic acid (Omega 6). Linolenic acid is converted in the body into DHA and EPA, which are also found in mackerel, herring, salmon, tuna and other fish. These essential fats are easily destroyed by heating or exposure to oxygen, so having a fresh daily source is important. Processed foods often contain hardened or 'hydrogenated' polyunsaturated fats. These are worse for you than saturated fat and are best avoided.

- **Eat** 1 tablespoon of cold-pressed seed oil (sesame, sunflower, pumpkin, flax seed, etc.) or 1 heaped tablespoon of ground seeds a day.

- **Avoid** fried food, burnt or browned fat, saturated and 'hydrogenated' fat.

Protein

Protein is made out of 22 amino acids, which are the building blocks of the body. As well as being vital for growth and the repair of body tissue, they are used to make hormones, enzymes, antibodies, neurotransmitters and help transport substances around the body. Both the quality of the protein you eat, determined by the balance of these amino acids, and the quantity you eat, are important.

In terms of quantity, the Government recommends that we obtain 15 per cent of our total calorie intake from protein, but gives little guidance as to the kind of protein. This is in sharp contrast to the average breast-fed baby, which receives just 1 per cent of its total calories from protein and manages to double its birth weight in 6 months. This is because the protein from breast milk is of very good quality and easily absorbed. Assuming good-quality protein, 10 per cent of calorie intake, or around 35 grams of protein a day, is an optimal intake for most people, unless pregnant, recovering from surgery or undertaking large amounts of exercise.

The best-quality protein foods in terms of amino acid balance include eggs, quinoa, soya, meat, fish, beans and lentils. Animal protein sources tend to contain a lot of undesirable saturated fat. Vegetable protein sources tend to contain additional beneficial complex carbohydrates and are less acid-forming than meat. It is best to limit eating meat to 3 times a week. In real terms it is difficult not to achieve adequate protein from any diet that includes 3 meals a day, whether they be vegan, vegetarian or meat-eating. Many vegetables, especially 'seed' foods like runner beans, peas, corn or broccoli, contain good levels of protein and help to neutralise excess acidity, which can lead to mineral losses including calcium, hence the higher risk of osteoporosis among frequent meat-eaters.

- **Eat** 2 servings of beans, lentils, quinoa, tofu (soya), 'seed' vegetables or other vegetable protein, or 1 small serving of meat, fish, cheese or a free-range egg a day.

- **Avoid** excess animal source protein.

Carbohydrate

Carbohydrate is the main fuel for the body. It comes in two forms: 'fast-releasing' – sugar, honey, malt, sweets and most refined foods – and 'slow-releasing', as in wholegrains, vegetables and fresh fruit. The latter foods contain more complex carbohydrate and/or more fibre, both of which help to slow down the release of sugar. Fast-releasing carbohydrates tend to give a sudden burst of energy, followed by a slump, while slow-releasing carbohydrates provide more sustained energy and are therefore preferable. Refined foods like sugar or white flour lack the vitamins and minerals needed for the body to use them properly and are best avoided. The perpetual use of fast-releasing carbohydrates can give rise to complex symptoms and health problems. Some fruits, like bananas, dates and raisins, contain faster-releasing sugars and are best kept to a minimum by people with glucose-related health problems (see Week 1, page 38). Slow-releasing carbohydrate foods – fresh fruit, vegetables, pulses and wholegrains - should make up two-thirds of what you eat, or around 70 per cent of your total calorie intake.

- **Eat** 3 or more servings of dark green, leafy and root vegetables such as watercress, carrots, sweet potatoes, broccoli, Brussels sprouts, spinach, green beans or peppers, raw or lightly cooked.

- **Eat** 3 or more servings of fresh fruit such as apples, pears, bananas, berries, melon or citrus fruit.

- **Eat** 4 or more servings of wholegrains such as rice, millet, rye, oats, wholewheat, corn, quinoa as cereal, breads, pasta or pulses.

- **Avoid** any form of sugar, foods with added sugar, white or refined foods.

Fibre

Rural Africans eat about 55 grams of dietary fibre a day, compared to the UK average intake of 22 grams. The ideal intake is not less than 35 grams a day. It is easy to get this amount of fibre – which absorbs water in the digestive tract, making the food contents bulkier and easier to pass through the body – by eating wholegrains, vegetables, fruit, nuts, seeds, lentils and beans on a daily basis. Fruit and vegetable fibre helps slow down the absorption of sugar into the blood, helping to maintain good energy levels. Cereal fibre is particularly good at preventing constipation and putrefaction of foods, which are underlying causes of many digestive complaints. Refined diets that are orientated towards meat, eggs, fish and dairy produce will undoubtedly lack fibre.

- **Eat** wholefoods – wholegrains, lentils, beans, nuts, seeds, fresh fruit and vegetables.

- **Avoid** refined, white and overcooked foods.

Water

Two-thirds of the body is made of water, which is therefore our most important nutrient. The body loses 1.5 litres of water a day through the skin, lungs and gut and via the kidneys as urine, ensuring that toxic substances are eliminated from the body. We also make about a third of a litre of water a day when glucose is 'burnt' for energy. Therefore, the minimum required water intake from food and drink is more than 1 litre a day and the ideal is around 2 litres.

Fruit and vegetables are around 90 per cent water, and provide it in a form that is very easy for the body to use, at the same time supplying the body with a high percentage of its vitamins and minerals. These foods can provide a litre of water, leaving 1 litre a day as an ideal intake, taken as water or in diluted juices, herb or fruit teas. Alcohol, tea and coffee cause the body to lose water, so are not recommended as sources of fluid intake. In addition, alcohol, tea and coffee rob the body of valuable minerals.

- **Drink** 1 litre of water a day as water or in diluted juices, herb or fruit teas.

- **Minimise** intake of alcohol, coffee or tea.

Vitamins

Vitamins are needed in much smaller amounts than fat, protein or carbohydrate but are no less important. They turn enzymes on, which in turn make all the body processes happen. Vitamins are needed to balance hormones, produce energy, boost the immune system, make healthy skin, protect the arteries, and are vital for the brain, nervous system and just about every body process. Vitamins A, C and E are antioxidants and keep you young by slowing down the ageing process and protecting the body from cancer, heart disease and pollution. B and C vitamins are vital for turning food into mental and physical energy. Vitamin D, found in milk, eggs, fish and meat, helps control calcium balance. It can also be made in the skin in the presence of sunshine. B and C vitamins are richest in living foods – fresh fruit and vegetables. Vitamin A comes in two forms: retinol, the animal form found in meat, fish, eggs and dairy produce; and beta-carotene, found in red, yellow and orange fruits and vegetables. Vitamin E is found in seeds, nuts and their oils and helps protect essential fats from going rancid.

- **Eat** 3 or more servings of dark green, leafy and root vegetables and 3 or more servings of fresh fruit plus some nuts or seeds every day.

- **Supplement** a multi-vitamin containing at least the following: vitamin A 2,250mcg, vitamin D 10mcg, vitamin E 100mg, vitamin B1 (thiamine) 25mg, B2 (riboflavin) 25mg, B3 (niacin) 50mg, B5 (pantothenic acid) 50mg, B6 50mg, B12 5mcg, folic acid 50mcg, biotin 50mcg. Also supplement 1,000mg of vitamin C a day.

Minerals

Minerals, like vitamins, are essential for just about every body process. Calcium, magnesium and phosphorus help make up the bones and teeth. Nerve signals, vital for the brain and muscles, depend on calcium, magnesium, sodium and potassium. Oxygen is carried in the blood by an iron compound. Chromium helps control blood sugar levels. Zinc is vital for all body repair, renewal and development. Selenium and zinc help boost the immune system. Brain function depends on adequate magnesium, manganese, zinc and other essential minerals. These are but a few out of thousands of key roles minerals play in human health. We need relatively large amounts of calcium and magnesium each day, and these are found in vegetables such as kale, cabbage and root vegetables as well as in nuts and seeds. Calcium alone is found in dairy produce. Fruits and vegetables also provide large amounts of potassium and small amounts of sodium, which is the right balance. All 'seed' foods, which include seeds, nuts, lentils and beans, as well as peas, broad beans, runner beans, wholegrains and even broccoli (the heads of which are the seeds), are good sources of iron, zinc, manganese and chromium. Seafood, seaweed and seeds, especially sesame, are rich in selenium.

- **Eat** 1 serving of mineral-rich foods such as kale, cabbage, root vegetables, low-fat dairy foods such as yoghurt, seeds or nuts such as almonds, as well as plenty of fresh fruit, vegetables and wholefoods such as lentils, beans and wholegrains.

- **Supplement** a multi-mineral containing at least the following: calcium 150mg, magnesium 75mg, iron 10mg, zinc 10mg, manganese 2.5mg, chromium 50mcg, selenium 25mcg.

Pure Food

Organic, unadulterated wholefoods have formed the basis of the human diet through the ages. Only now in the twentieth century has the human race been subjected to countless man-made chemicals found in food and the environment.

One foundation of health is to eat foods that provide exactly the amount of energy required to keep the body in perfect balance. A good deal of energy is wasted trying to disarm these alien and often toxic chemicals, some of which cannot be eliminated and accumulate in body tissue. It is now impossible to avoid all such substances, as there is nowhere on this planet that is not contaminated in some way from the by-products of our modern chemical age. Choosing organic foods whenever possible is the nearest we can get to eating a pure diet today. By supporting the movement back to pure, organic food we help to minimise the damage of chemical pollution, which poses a real threat to the future of humanity.

Raw, organic food is the most natural and beneficial way to take food into the body. Many foods contain enzymes that help our bodies digest them once the food is chewed. Raw food is full of vital phytochemicals whose effect on our health may prove as important as vitamins and minerals. Cooking food destroys enzymes and can reduce the activity of phytochemicals.

- **Eat** organic as much as possible. Make sure at least half your diet is raw fruit, vegetables, wholegrains, nuts and seeds.

- **Avoid** processed food with lists of additives and cook foods as little as possible.

Top 10 Diet Tips

Here are 10 top tips for transforming your daily diet for better health:

1 heaped tablespoon of ground seeds or 1 tablespoon of cold-pressed seed oil.
2 servings of beans, lentils, quinoa, tofu (soya), or 'seed' vegetables.
3 pieces of fresh fruit such as apples, pears, bananas, berries, melon or citrus fruit.
4 servings of wholegrains such as rice, millet, rye, oats, wholewheat, corn, quinoa as cereal, breads or pasta.
5 servings of dark green, leafy and root vegetables such as watercress, carrots, sweet potatoes, broccoli, spinach, green beans, peas and peppers.
6 glasses of water, diluted juices, herb or fruit teas.
7 Eat whole, organic, raw food as much as you can.
8 Supplement a high-strength multi-vitamin and mineral and 1,000 mg of vitamin C a day.
9 Avoid fried, burnt or browned food, 'hydrogenated' fat and excess animal fat.
10 Avoid any form of sugar, white, refined or processed food with chemical additives and minimise your intake of alcohol, coffee or tea – maximum 1 alcoholic drink a day.

BASIC PRINCIPLE 2

Supplements for Superhealth

Supplements are an essential part of a superhealth strategy. Even if you eat all the right foods you are unlikely to achieve an optimal intake of all vitamins and minerals.

Through these 6 Weeks to Superhealth I recommend that you take a good multi-vitamin and multi-mineral supplement and additional vitamin C, providing, at least, the following amounts of vitamins and minerals:

A multi-vitamin containing at least the following:

vitamin A	2,250mcg
vitamin D	10mcg
vitamin E	100mg
vitamin B1 (thiamine)	25mg
B2 (riboflavin)	25mg
B3 (niacin)	50mg
B5 (pantothenic acid)	50mg
B6	50mg
B12	5mcg
folic acid	50mcg
biotin	50mcg

A multi-mineral containing at least the following:

calcium	150mg
magnesium	75mg
iron	10mg
zinc	10mg
manganese	2.5mg
chromium	50mcg
selenium	25mcg

A vitamin C supplement providing 1,000mg vitamin C

In addition to these basic supplements, other supplements are added to each of the 6 weeks to support the objective of that section of the programme. For example, in Week 1, when you'll be focusing on balancing your blood sugar, I recommend that you also supplement 200mcg of the mineral chromium. Some supplements, such as chromium, are continued throughout the 6 weeks (or at least until you finish the tub). Others, such as the digestive enzyme supplement in the second week, are just taken for the relevant week. While there is no problem continuing to take each additional supplement, you may end up taking more supplements than you really need – you will soon see what works best for you and if you find the addition of a specific supplement to be especially beneficial, by all means keep taking it. Otherwise a qualified clinical nutritionist can help you work out your personal needs (see Support and Resources, page 216).

In each week there are also 'optional' supplements that you can add if you are dealing with a specific problem. For example, in Week 2, which focuses on digestion, if you have particular problems in this area you can also add colon-cleansing herbs and fibres.

Exactly which supplements you need to buy, and where you can get them from, is detailed on pages 213–15 so you can get stocked up before you start.

BASIC PRINCIPLE 3

Exercising for Superhealth

No superhealth programme would be complete without stressing the importance of exercise. The exercise system that I strongly recommend is called *Psychocalisthenics*. It is easy to learn and the results are better than any other exercise regime I've come across. Oscar Ichazo, originator of *Psychocalisthenics*, believes that, 'As promoters of health, normally only two fundamental parameters are analysed: diet and exercise. But we forget or ignore the other basic element that is vital energy, not to be confused with vitality, which is the healthy result of the three parameters (diet, exercise, and vital energy) in balance.'

Psychocalisthenics, which is a routine of 23 exercises that can be done in less than 20 minutes, is a complete contemporary exercise system which, at first glance, looks like a powerful kind of aerobic yoga. 'In the same way that we have an everyday need for food and nourishment we have to promote the circulation of our vital energy as an everyday business,' says Ichazo, who has studied and practised martial arts and yoga since 1939, as well as founding the Arica School in the 1960s as a school of knowledge for the understanding of the complete man.

Psychocalisthenics is the unity of the body and mind across the breath. The breath is the driving force in this routine, as each of the 23 exercises is guided by a precise deep breathing pattern. This combination of movement, breath and exercises, designed to generate vital energy, is what makes *Psychocalisthenics* unique – a perfect combination of East and West. When I first learnt the routine I was amazed at how light and re-energised my body felt afterwards. My muscles felt tuned, my joints more flexible, but the major benefit was this feeling of clear-headedness. Other advocates of *Psychocalisthenics* give the same glowing reports. 'This is exercise pared to perfection. I wasn't sweating buckets as I would after an aerobics class but I could feel I had exercised far more muscles. I was feeling clear-headed and bright rather than wiped out,' said Jane Alexander, when she reviewed the routine for the *Daily Mail*. In the US, *Psychocalisthenics* is now promoted by the 'bionic woman', actress Lindsay Wagner.

While most exercise routines simply treat the body as a physical machine that needs to be worked to stay fit, *Psychocalisthenics* is designed to generate both physical fitness and vital energy by bringing the mind and body into balance. The key lies in the precise breathing pattern than accompanies each physical exercise. 'Once we integrate our mind with our body across a controlled respiration, we can produce in ourselves an element of self-observation that is indispensable for acquiring understanding of our true nature,' says Ichazo. 'What *Psychocalisthenics* offers is a set of exercises that can become a serious foundation for a life of self-responsibility, clarity of mind, and strength of spirit.'

One of the things I like most about *Psychocalisthenics* is that you don't have to go anywhere, or wear special clothes, or buy any equipment.

Quick-Reference Chart for *Psychocalisthenics*

Each of your **6 Weeks to Superhealth** introduces 3 or more of the 23 *Psychocalisthenics* exercises for you to practise every day. Each week you'll learn and add on a new set of exercises until, by Week 6, you'll be doing the whole routine (listed below for quick reference). But before you start make sure you follow and master the instructions for the exercises that are given week by week in Part 3 (page 37).

Week 1
Integration Breath ✕3
Picking Grapes ✕6
Integration Breath ✕1
Lateral Stretch ✕6
Integration Breath ✕1
Flamingo ✕6

Week 2
All the above plus . . .
Integration Breath ✕1
Ax 1 ✕6
Ax 2 ✕3
Integration Breath ✕1
Udiyama ✕3

Week 3
All the above plus . . .
Integration Breath ✕1
Shoulder Rolls ✕6
Integration Breath ✕1
Arm Circles ✕6
Integration Breath ✕1
Hand Circles ✕6
Integration Breath ✕1

Week 4
All the above plus . . .
Windmill ✕3
Integration Breath ✕1
Scythe ✕6
Integration Breath ✕1
Head Circles left ✕6, right ✕6
Side-to-side ✕6
Camel ✕6
Lung Breath ✕3

Week 5
All the above plus . . .
Candle/Plough ✕3
Bow ✕6
Leg Circles ✕6
Scissors ✕6

Week 6
All the above plus . . .
Cobra ✕3
Integration Breath ✕1
Pendulum ✕9 each leg
Integration Breath ✕3
Completo ✕1
Integration Breath ✕3
Completo ✕1
Integration Breath ✕3

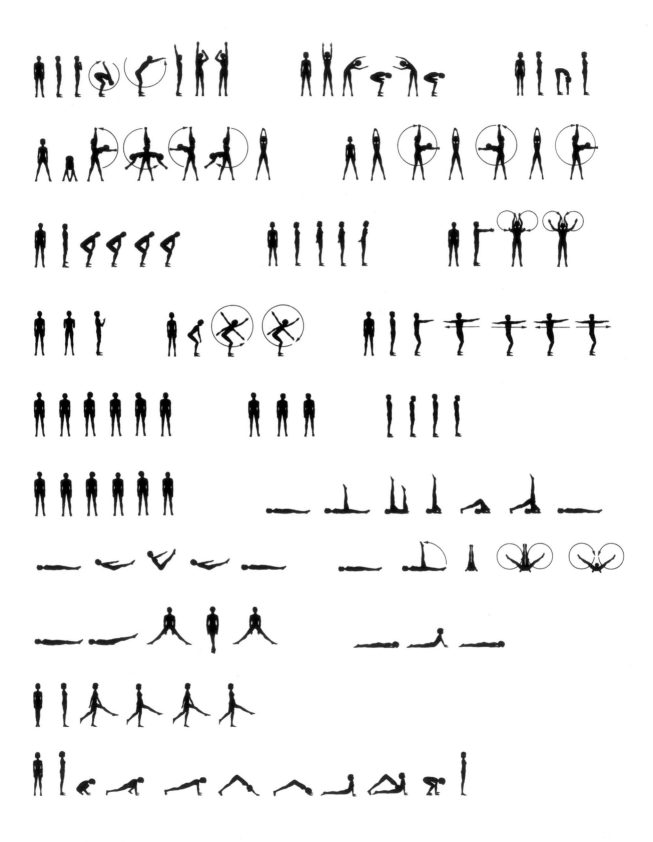

What You Need to Know

Study the diagrams which show the movements in the entire sequence of exercises. The instructions for each exercise are given week by week in Part 3 (page 37). The number of times each exercise is to be repeated is shown as, for example, '×3' (three times). Once you have learned *Psychocalisthenics*, concentrate on making the movements smooth and rhythmical. Be aware of the different parts of the body being worked by each exercise. Do the entire workout for each week in one session on a regular basis. The best time to do *Psychocalisthenics* is shortly after you wake up. Doing too much too quickly may result in soreness and strain.

Principles

With *Psychocalisthenics*, the result you get is proportional to how carefully you practise the exercises. Important points of attention are the position of the feet, the pattern of breathing, concentration in the *Kath* (balance point), and relaxation. Perform *Psychocalisthenics* with an attitude of enthusiasm and motivation.

- **Foot positions** The foot position specified in each diagram provides stability and balance. The outsides of the feet are kept parallel. The distance between your feet is measured in foot-widths. Use your feet to measure each position accurately.

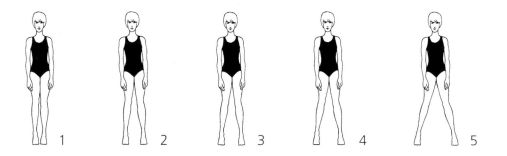

1. Position of equilibrium: Feet flush against each other.

2. Position of movement: Feet parallel, 1–1½ foot-widths apart.

3. Standing position: Feet parallel, 2 foot-widths apart.

4. Position of strength: Feet parallel, 3 foot-widths apart. This is approximately shoulder-width.

5. Position of relaxation: Feet parallel, 5 foot-widths apart. This is the farthest apart the feet can be placed without breaking the arch formed by the legs and the pelvis.

Having feet parallel means that the second toes point straight ahead. This may feel pigeon-toed at first.

- **Breathing** A precise pattern of breathing is given for each exercise. This supports the expansion and contraction of the lungs when you move and integrates the body with the entire exercise. Synchronize the breathing pattern with your movements as shown in the diagrams. The black arrows indicate inhalation; the white arrows indicate exhalation. The arrows also show the direction of the movement. Throughout the sequence, inhale through your nose and exhale through your mouth. Inhale and exhale completely.

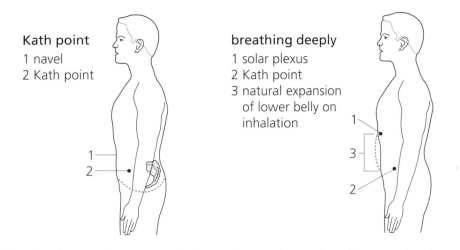

Kath point
1 navel
2 Kath point

breathing deeply
1 solar plexus
2 Kath point
3 natural expansion of lower belly on inhalation

Go for the maximum ventilation of your lungs, breathing as deeply as possible without strain.

- **Concentration in the Kath** Maintain concentration in your *Kath* (balance point), located 3 finger-widths below your navel. This increases the kinesthetic awareness of your body. Dia-Kath breathing, the Awareness Exercise in Week 1, will help you to develop this deeper method of breathing.

- **Relaxation** Perform *Psychocalisthenics* in a relaxed fashion. The vital energy generated by the movements and breathing flows throughout your entire body when you are relaxed. Do not lock your knees but keep them relaxed.

- **Learning *Psychocalisthenics*** Once you've learnt the routine you can do it in 16 minutes in your own home, accompanied either by the video, or with a 'talk through' tape of synchronised music. The best way to learn it is to do a one-day training (details on training are given on page 217). You can also learn it from the video, but there's nothing like having someone there to tell you what you're doing wrong and how to do it right. There's a fascinating book by Oscar Ichazo called *Master Level Exercise, Psychocalisthenics*, which explains the theory behind *Psychocalisthenics* and how each exercise revitalises different parts of the body and mind (see page 217).

A word of warning Consult your doctor before attempting this or any other exercise routine, especially if you have a history of back or heart problems, or are pregnant. The author, publisher, and distributors of this book disclaim any liability or loss in connection with the exercises or material contained within.

BASIC PRINCIPLE 4

Psyched Up for Superhealth

Superhealth isn't just a state of the body, it's a state of the body and mind. Disease is more often than not the consequence of mind and body working in opposition. After all, it is a mind which is not at ease that makes us over-exert ourselves or become anxious which tenses the body, or depressed which suppresses immunity, or consume excess food or alcohol to numb situations we find uncomfortable. We create our own internal reality which, often different from actual reality, leaves us in a state of 'dis-ease'.

The right attitude for superhealth is one of being in reality, of being aware of the needs of the body and bringing the mind and body into harmony. For this reason, each week of your 6 Weeks to Superhealth includes simple awareness exercises that will help you reconnect with your body's needs. For example, there are relaxation exercises, breathing exercises, exercises to help you nourish yourself more consciously by chewing your food, exercises to help you understand what you do to lose energy and what you can do to gain it. In fact, everything in these 6 weeks, from the diet to the physical exercises, will make you so much more conscious of your mental, emotional and physical needs. It will give you an experience of being grounded and centred in your self, no longer with your mind and body pulling in different directions.

To get the most out of these 6 weeks it is best to embrace this time as a real opportunity to change, to bring yourself back into balance and to experience a new level of energy. Use this time as a retreat. In addition to following the guidelines, plan your 6 weeks to support your experience of superhealth. For example, do other exercises, go for walks, spend weekends in the country, take time off, read inspirational books, see uplifting movies, don't work too hard, get enough sleep, pace yourself. Spend time with good friends who will support you in carrying out the superhealth strategy and spend some time alone. Best of all, encourage your friends to embark on 6 Weeks to Superhealth together so you can support each other. If you are drawn to any spiritual practices or exercises, such as meditation, yoga or tai chi, include these in your 6 weeks. If there are any addictions you wish to quit, such as smoking, this is a great time to do it.

Also, put your full intention behind following the instructions to the letter. Make that easy for yourself by shopping in advance so you have all the foods and supplements you need. Simultaneously, give your kitchen a spring-clean and get rid of all the junk food in your fridge and cupboards so you won't be tempted. Inevitably, there may be situations where you are tempted to break the rules – for example if you're invited out to dinner to celebrate a birthday and there's nothing on the menu that quite fits! There are two choices: either ask for something simple that's not on the menu, like a simple fish dish with vegetables, or bend the rules and get back on track the next day. If you do deviate from the diet, notice how you feel. During these 6 weeks you will become increasingly sensitive about the effects different foods have on you.

Getting Ready

So now you are ready to get started. Here's what to do:

- **Go food shopping for the week** There's a shopping list on page 212. Look at the recommended recipes for the week and add any ingredients for them to your shopping list.

- **Stock up with supplements** There's a list of what you need on page 213, with suggestions on specific products and where you can get them. If you live in a country where access to more specialised supplements is limited you may need to order some by mail-order or on the web. Most mail-order companies are used to sending supplements abroad.

- **Learn *Psychocalisthenics*** Each week of the 6 Weeks to Superhealth programme gives you the indications for each exercise, so if you follow the instructions carefully you can easily learn the whole routine, adding 3 or 4 exercises each week until you are completing the entire series of 23 exercises. If you require further information I have included details of training days, videos, tapes and supporting literature on page 217.

- **Prepare your space** For *Psychocalisthenics* you will need a well-ventilated space, 6ft by 6ft, and a carpet or mat for the floor exercises. For some of the Awareness Exercises you will also need somewhere quiet where you can sit or lie down. You may wish to create an area where you can do these exercises. Also, clean up your kitchen and make a space for your supplements.

- **Set aside time** All this exercise and food preparation takes time so you may want to think about reorganising your day and establishing a routine. Here's an example:

Morning Routine

7.30am	Wake Up
7.30–7.40am	*Psychocalisthenics*
7.40–7.50am	Awareness Exercise (as appropriate – some happen throughout the day)
7.50–8.05am	Shower, get dressed
8.05–8.30am	Breakfast, take supplements, prepare lunch

Evening Routine

6.30–6.40pm	Awareness Exercise (as appropriate)
6.40–7.30pm	Prepare and eat dinner, take supplements

Now you have grasped the basic principles of superhealth you are ready to embark on the 6-week programme. Work through the next 6 sections, one section per week, until you've completed the course. If you feel that one area of your health needs special attention, I recommend that you repeat the relevant week.

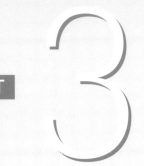

PART 3

6 WEEKS TO SUPERHEALTH

1 Supercharge Your Energy ✓

2 Tune Up Your Digestion ✓

3 Balance Your Hormones ✓

4 Detox for Superhealth ✓

5 Boost Your Immune Power ✓

6 Improve Your Memory and Mood ✓

WEEK 1

SUPERCHARGE YOUR ENERGY

Making Energy

We are solar-powered. That is, the energy in our food comes from the sun. Plants use the sun's energy to combine water from the soil and carbon dioxide from the air to make carbohydrate. We eat the plant, break the carbohydrate down into glucose and release the sun's energy contained within it.

Almost all of the body's energy is derived from glucose – sugar. This is the main 'fuel' of the body and what you eat determines the quality, the quantity and the availability of glucose to all your body's cells, including the brain. Consequently, maintaining an even blood sugar level is of paramount importance with regard to energy, mood and overall health. A key way to control this is by what you eat, especially the type of carbohydrate.

All carbohydrates are broken down by digestion into sugar, which is released into the bloodstream to provide the entire body with fuel. The mechanisms by which this works have an effect on our energy, mood, weight, our ability to deal with stress and our long-term health.

Most of us are sub-optimally nourished. This means that our body cells cannot make energy efficiently so the first sign of sub-optimum nutrition is fatigue. This is nothing new. Throughout history fatigue and stress have existed and man has searched for ways to banish both. This has led to the isolation of 'stimulants' which are chemicals that give you a boost – such as tea, coffee, cigarettes, chocolate and sugar.

Stimulants give your energy a boost by stimulating the adrenal glands. These glands, situated on top of the kidneys, release hormones that initiate express delivery of energy-giving glucose to cells. Such 'express delivery' is much more expensive than regular mail, and leads to both a deficiency in key nutrients and fluctuating blood sugar and energy levels. This is why you may experience a dip in energy and concentration a few hours after taking in stimulants.

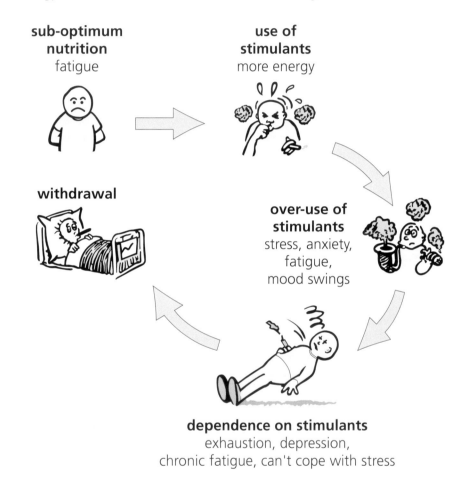

sub-optimum nutrition
fatigue

use of stimulants
more energy

withdrawal

over-use of stimulants
stress, anxiety, fatigue, mood swings

dependence on stimulants
exhaustion, depression, chronic fatigue, can't cope with stress

The vicious circle of stress and fatigue

The addictive nature of stimulants is their downside. That's why occasional use of stimulants leads to regular use of stimulants and, in due course, as your body's chemistry gets more and more exhausted, you need even more of the stimulant to get the same effect. By now you're a coffee connoisseur, can't function without that cup of tea or are addicted to chocolate or cigarettes.

Our bodies have only a finite capacity to detoxify undesirable substances. Excessive intake of sugar and stimulants, coupled with sub–optimum nutrition, starts to overload the body's detoxification potential, and once you've exceeded this adaptive capacity your ability to cope with the otherwise normal stresses of modern living becomes compromised.

The road to recovery requires some major dietary and lifestyle changes. As a result of the body's lack of health reserve, it becomes necessary, for a while, to completely clean up your act. This means avoiding as much as possible all stimulants and toxic substances, focusing on taking into the body only highly nutritious foods plus high levels of key nutrients by taking specific nutritional supplements.

Once you've built up a good health reserve it isn't necessary to be quite so saint-like all of the time. A strong body can cope with an infrequent indulgence. At this stage you are in such a condition that very often your body will let you know quickly if something you're doing isn't suiting you. Now, with extra awareness based on your experience, you'll be less inclined to 'over-ride' your body's warning signals and more likely to avoid another vicious cycle of stress and fatigue.

To get to grips with this cycle and know how to avoid it or recover from it, we need to delve deeper into how the body makes and maintains energy. Its primary fuel is carbohydrate (made up of sugar): balancing your blood sugar level is critical to maintaining a high energy level and an ability to cope with stress.

How the Body Stores Energy

If the only way your body could get glucose was directly from food you'd be dead in two days if you stopped eating. When you run out of glucose the body breaks down glycogen (stored in the liver and in muscles) into glucose. When glycogen stores are used up the body burns fat. When fat stores are used up the body burns lean tissue. Conversely, if your blood glucose level is fine and your glycogen stores are full, the body stores the fat you eat as fat. If you eat carbo-hydrate your body digests this down to glucose. If your blood glucose level is fine, the liver soaks up this glucose like a sponge and converts it to glycogen. If your glycogen stores are full, it's converted to fat.

So your ability to maintain an even blood sugar level depends not only on what you eat, but also on how efficient your body is at keeping everything in

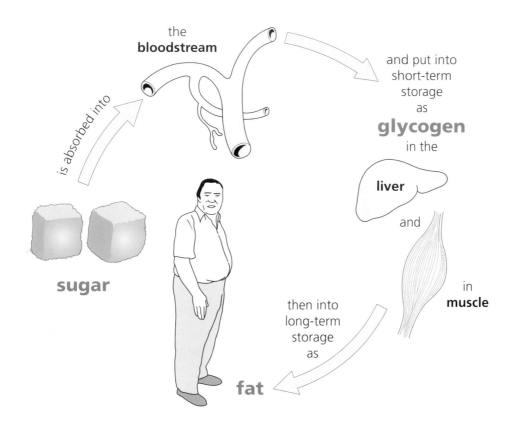

How the body stores energy as fat

balance by putting excess glucose into storage and, at times of shortage, raiding your energy reserves.

Since every single cell in your body runs on glucose, when there's a shortage not only does your body get physically tired, so too does your mind. You get forgetful, lose your concentration and can't think straight. Emotionally you get irritable, depressed and less able to cope. Such symptoms are everyday occurrences for many people, who, for one reason or another, lose their ability to keep their blood sugar level even and become over-sensitive to its highs and lows. This is technically called dysglycaemia, or sugar sensitivity, and is thought to affect about 1 in 4 people.

The 3 big baddies as far as blood sugar is concerned are sugar, stimulants and stress. On the next few pages you will find some questionnaires which will help you discover to what degree sugar, stress and stimulants may be affecting your life. When you have worked through the questionnaires, read on to discover what your next move should be. First, you need to check your energy levels.

Week 1

CHECK YOUR ENERGY

Complete this questionnaire to discover whether your energy levels are slumping because you are sugar sensitive.

	C	T
Are you barely wide awake within 20 minutes of rising?	N	N
Do you need tea, coffee, a cigarette or something to get you going in the morning?	Y	N
Do you really like sweet foods?	Y	Y
Do you crave bread, cereal, popcorn or pasta?	Y	N
Do you feel like you 'need' an alcoholic drink on most days?	N	N
Are you overweight and unable to shift the extra pounds?	N	N
Do you often have energy slumps during the day or after meals?	Y	N
Do you often have mood swings or difficulty concentrating?	Y	N
Do you get dizzy or irritable if you go 6 hours without food?	Y	N
Do you often find you over-react to stress?	Y	N
Do you often get irritable, angry or aggressive unexpectedly?	Y	N
Is your energy now less than it used to be?	Y	Y
Do you feel you could never give up bread?	N	N
Do you suffer from continual hunger?	N	N
Do you suffer from depression?	N	Y

- If you answer 'yes' to 7 or more questions there's a very good chance that you are sugar sensitive and struggling to keep your blood sugar level even.

- If you answer 'yes' to between 4 and 7 questions you are beginning to show signs of a sugar sensitivity which needs to be redressed.

- If you answer 'yes' to less than 4 questions, you are unlikely to have a blood sugar problem.

Week 1

Sugar – the Sweet Truth

Eating too much sugar and refined carbohydrates not only zaps your energy – it has many harmful effects on your health. Glucose is highly toxic. That's why the body tries to get it out of the blood as quickly as possible. Too much glucose damages the arteries, kidneys, eyes and nerves, which is what often happens in people with diabetes.

The association between high sugar, refined carbohydrate and an increased risk of cardiovascular disease is well established. When blood sugar levels rise, the excess glucose immediately starts to damage proteins found in the arteries.

Sugar can also make you fat. This is because the more frequently your blood sugar is raised, the more insulin you produce. The more insulin you produce, the more sugar you dump as fat. Sugar can not only lead to weight gain and obesity, but also to water retention. If your body is too full of sugar you'll retain excess fluid too, as every molecule of sugar will hold water.

Sugar can also greatly affect moods and anyone who suffers from depression, PMS, hyperactivity, irritability, mood swings or angry outbursts should examine whether they are having a problem controlling their blood sugar.

It is easy to become reliant on a daily intake of sugar, and if the thought of stopping sugar overnight makes you shudder you may well want to consider whether you are addicted. Later in Week 1 we'll be looking at ways to deal with this.

ARE YOU A SUGAR ADDICT?

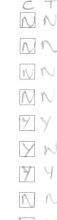

- Do you ever lie about how much sweet food you have eaten?
- Do you keep a supply of sweet food close to hand?
- Have you ever hidden your supply from others?
- Have you ever got upset if someone else ate your sweet food?
- Have you ever gone out of your way to buy sweet foods?
- Do you eat sweet foods when you are emotionally upset?
- Do you swoon at the dessert menu and take a mint on the way out?
- Do you think a lot about and look forward to your sugary 'treat'?
- Do you think you are addicted to sugar, chocolate or biscuits?

If you answer 'yes' 5 or more times consider yourself a sugar addict.

Week 1

Are You Addicted to Stress?

Body chemistry fundamentally changes every time a person reacts to stress. Stress starts in the mind. We perceive a situation as requiring our immediate attention – a young child getting too close to the road, a hostile reaction from someone – and rapid signals stimulate the adrenal glands (situated on top of the kidneys in the small of the back) to produce adrenalin. Within seconds our heart is pounding, our breathing changes, stores of glucose are released into the blood, the muscles tense, the eyes dilate, the blood thickens. This gets us ready to 'fight or take flight' – our ancestors may have had a use for this, but now the average adrenalin rush of a commuter stuck in a traffic jam is enough to keep him running for a mile. That's how much glucose is released, mainly by breaking down glycogen held in muscles and the liver.

To get the fuel into body cells, the pancreas releases 2 hormones, insulin and glucagon. Insulin helps carry the fuel out of the blood and into the cells; glucagon tops up the blood sugar if levels get too low. Another substance, released from the liver, Glucose Tolerance Factor, potentiates the effect of insulin. All this is happening as a result of a stressful thought. Imagine your pituitary and adrenal glands, pancreas and liver perpetually pumping out hormones to control blood sugar that you don't even need, day in, day out. Like a car driven too fast, the body goes out of balance and parts start to wear out.

ARE YOU STRESSING YOURSELF OUT?

C   T

- Is your energy less now than it used to be?   ☑ Y
- Do you feel guilty when relaxing?   ☑ Y
- Do you have a persistent need for achievement?   ☑ Y
- Are you unclear about your goals in life?   ☑ N
- Are you especially competitive?   ☑ Y
- Do you work harder than most people?   ☑ Y
- Do you easily become angry?   ☑ N
- Do you often do 2 or 3 tasks simultaneously?   ☑ Y
- Do you get impatient if people or things hold you up?   ☑ Y
- Do you have difficulty getting to sleep?   ☑ N

If you answer 'yes' 5 or more times you're in the high stress category.

Instead of using these stress hormones as a back-up, a supercharge only to be used in times of emergency, many of us live permanently on adrenalin and other stress hormones, going from one stress to another, living off coffee, tea, cigarettes or sugar. After a while it's only the adrenalin that keeps us going. If you quit the stimulants or take some time off, you collapse into a heap – depressed and exhausted. This means that you've become addicted to stress or stimulants. Later in Week 1 we'll be looking at how you can deal with your stress levels.

You Don't Need Stimulants

Stimulants are energy's greatest enemy. Even though stimulants can create energy in the short term, the long-term effect is always bad. Imagine a day with no coffee, tea, sugar, chocolate, cigarettes or alcohol. If the thought of this is intolerable, you have an addiction to stimulants. It's worth knowing what each of these stimulants contains and what their effect is on the body.

- **Alcohol** is made by the action of yeast on sugar. As such it has a similar effect to sugar. In the short term alcohol actually inhibits the release of reserve glucose from the liver and encourages low blood sugar levels, causing an increase in appetite.

- **Chocolate** contains cocoa as its major 'active' ingredient. Cocoa provides significant quantities of the stimulant theobromine, whose action is similar to, although not as strong as, caffeine.

- **Cigarettes** contain nicotine, as well as 16 other cancer-producing chemicals. Nicotine is the primary stimulant and has a substantial effect even in small doses. In large amounts, nicotine acts as a sedative. It is more addictive than heroin.

- **Coffee** contains theobromine, theophylline and caffeine, all of which are stimulants. Caffeine is the major stimulant, but decaffeinated coffee still contains the other two. Theophylline disturbs normal sleep patterns. Coffee consumption is associated with greater risk of cancer of the pancreas.

- **Cola** drinks can contain a quarter of the caffeine found in a weak cup of coffee. They usually contain sugar and colourings which can also act as stimulants.

- **Medication** for the relief of headaches may contain caffeine. Other caffeine tablets and drinks are available as stimulants. The most common are Pro Plus, Red Bull and the herb Guarana.

- **Tea** contains caffeine, theobromine, theophylline and tannin. It is a stimulant and a diuretic, with similar, although lesser, effects to coffee. A strong cup of tea can provide as much caffeine as a weak cup of coffee. Tannin interferes with the absorption of minerals. Tea drinkers have an increased risk of stomach ulcers.

In making an assessment of your current relationship to stimulants it is very helpful to get real about your actual intake.

STIMULANT CHECK

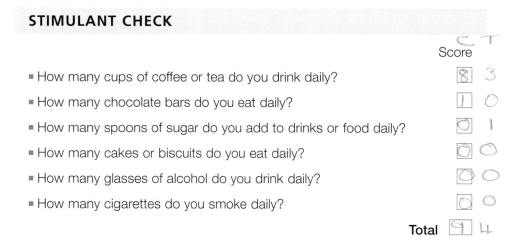

Score

- How many cups of coffee or tea do you drink daily?   8   3
- How many chocolate bars do you eat daily?   1   0
- How many spoons of sugar do you add to drinks or food daily?   0   1
- How many cakes or biscuits do you eat daily?   0   0
- How many glasses of alcohol do you drink daily?   0   0
- How many cigarettes do you smoke daily?   0   0

Total   9   4

If you score more than 7, the chances are that you are a stimulant addict.

Balancing Blood Sugar

Now you've established why your energy levels are so low you need to do something about it. There are 3 main ways to keep the levels stable and to overcome the influence of (or addiction to) those 3 baddies – sugar, stress and stimulants:

1. Increase slow-releasing carbohydrates in your diet.

2. Reduce your stress and stimulants.

3. Introduce energy nutrients.

1 Increase Slow-releasing Carbohydrates

The first way to increase your energy levels is via your carbohydrate intake. Some carbohydrates are 'fast-releasing' in that they raise blood sugar quickly, while others are 'slow-releasing'. The fast-releasing foods are like rocket fuel – they give a quick burst of energy with a rapid burn-out. It is important to choose foods which are 'slow-releasing' as they are much more sustaining, giving a consistent energy level throughout the day. What makes a food slow- or fast-releasing depends on many factors. Foods contain different kinds of sugars. Wholegrains, for example, such as wholemeal pasta, rice and breads, are rich in slow-releasing sugars. Most fruits are rich in slow-releasing fructose – fruit sugar. Sweets and sweet foods contain fast-releasing sucrose or glucose which shoot the blood sugar up too quickly, giving us that consequent slump. Stimulants and stress have similar effects on the blood sugar. This is where addictions can raise their ugly heads, keeping us reaching for those sugary foods, or stimulants, giving ourselves a quick energy 'fix' as we reach that slump. Therefore to keep sustained, high levels of energy throughout the day, it is important to avoid sugar, stress and stimulants as well as choosing the right energy foods.

But how do you know what is fast- or slow-releasing? The very measure of a food's fast- or slow-releasing effect is linked to the degree to which it raises your blood sugar: this can be worked out on a scale called the glycaemic index (GI for short). It involves measuring the level to which a food raises your blood glucose in relation to the effect glucose has (see page 49). If a food raises blood sugar levels significantly, and for some time, the area under the curve made by glucose is great. Conversely if a food hardly raises blood sugar levels at all, and only for a short time, the area under the curve is small. The curve created by glucose, the fastest-releasing sugar, is given a value of 100, and other foods are scored in relation to this. If a food creates a curve with half the area it measures 50. The amount of food tested obviously affects how high the blood sugar level will go. Here, we've used a usual serving size of a food to indicate its relative effect on your blood sugar.

The chart on page 48 gives the GI score of an average serving of common foods. Check out what you eat for breakfast. If you start your day with raisins and puffed rice cereal, both of which have a high GI score, you're setting yourself up for a rapid burn-out. On the other hand, kick off with oat flakes, sweetened with a chopped apple, both of which are slow-releasing, and your energy will last for longer.

The Glycaemic Index of Common Foods

Food	Score	Food	Score	Food	Score
Sugars		*Breads and biscuits*		*Dairy products/substitutes*	
Glucose	100	French baguette	95	Tofu ice cream	73
Maltose	100	Rice cake	82	Ice cream (low fat)	50
Honey	87	Wholemeal crispbread	81	Yoghurt	36
Sucrose (sugar)	59	Water biscuit	76	Whole milk	34
Fructose (fruit sugar)	20	Waffle	76	Skimmed milk	32
		Bagel	72		
Fruit		White bread	70	*Vegetables*	
Watermelon	72	Wholemeal bread	69	Parsnips (cooked)	97
Pineapple	66	Ryvita	69	Potato (baked)	85
Melon	65	Crumpet	69	Potato (instant)	80
Raisins	64	Digestive biscuits	59	Broad beans	79
Banana	62	Pitta bread	57	Pumpkin (boiled)	75
Apricots (fresh)	57	Sourdough rye bread	57	French fries	75
Kiwi fruit	52	Rich tea biscuits	55	Potato (new, boiled)	70
Grapes	46	Oatmeal biscuits	54	Beetroot (cooked)	64
Orange	40	Wholegrain wheat bread	46	Sweetcorn	59
Apple	39	Wholegrain rye bread	41	Sweet potato	54
Plum	39			Peas	51
Pear	38	*Cereals*		Carrots (cooked)	49
Apricots (dried)	30	Cornflakes	80		
Grapefruit	25	Puffed rice	73	*Snacks and drinks*	
Cherries	25	Weetabix	69	Lucozade	95
		Shredded wheat	67	Pretzels	83
Grains and grain products		Muesli	66	Jelly beans	80
White rice	72	Kellogg's Special K	54	Corn chips	72
Taco shells	68	Kellogg's All-Bran	52	Fanta	68
Brown rice	66	Porridge oats	49	Mars Bar	68
Couscous	65			Squash (diluted)	66
Bran muffin	60	*Pulses*		Muesli bar with fruit	65
Basmati rice	58	Baked beans	48	Muesli bar	61
Buckwheat	54	Baked beans (no sugar)	40	Popcorn (low fat)	55
Apple muffin	54	Butter beans	36	Potato crisps	54
Pastry	50	Chickpeas	36	Orange juice	46
White spaghetti	50	Black-eyed beans	33	Apple juice	40
Instant noodles	46	Haricot beans	31	Peanuts	14
Wholemeal spaghetti	42	Kidney beans	29		
Barley	26	Lentils	29		
		Soya beans	15		

Some of these figures may be surprising, and we can begin to see how re-thinking areas of our diet can help our blood sugar levels.

Generally, foods with a GI score below 50 are great to include in your diet, while those with a score above 70 should be avoided or mixed with a low-scoring food. Those with a score between 50 and 70 should be eaten infrequently and only with a low-scoring food. For example, bananas are quite high, with a score of 62. Oat flakes and skimmed milk are low, with a score of 49 and 32 respectively. Having a bowl of oat flakes with skimmed milk and half a banana for breakfast would help to keep your blood sugar level on an even keel, while eating cornflakes (scoring 80) with raisins (scoring 64) would be bad news.

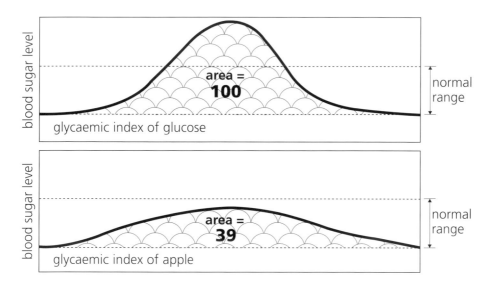

Measuring the Glycaemic Index of a food

2 Reduce Your Stress and Stimulants

These 2 baddies often come hand in hand, perpetuating the 'addiction' cycle. Stimulants can keep the body constantly stressed, so it is important to work on reducing them both to break the habit cycle completely. Look at your life and identify where your main stressors lie in order to begin the process of de-stressing. For example, identify how you expend energy and develop better ways to respond and deal with stressful situations. Include some form of de-stressing exercise in your weekly routine such as *Psychocalisthenics*, yoga or tai chi, and put aside some time for meditation, contemplation or getting away from it all. Go for walks in the country or by the sea. And do get enough sleep, ideally 7 hours a night.

It is important to replace your regular stimulant with 'alternatives' that you actually like – so experiment. Remember that when you break your habit, and your blood sugar begins to level out, the cravings will disappear and you will begin to really enjoy these alternatives. Check out what's available in your healthfood shop.

- **Coffee** is strongly addictive. It takes, on average, 4 days to break the habit. During these days you may experience headaches and grogginess. These are a strong reminder of how bad coffee really is for you. Decaffeinated coffee is only slightly better. The most popular coffee alternatives are Caro, Dandex, Barleycup, Yannoh and Symington's Dandelion Coffee.

- **Tea** is not as bad for you as coffee, unless you're the sort of person that likes your tea well stewed. Use Luaka tea, which is a good quality Ceylon tea that is naturally low in tannin and caffeine. The most popular alternatives are herb and fruit teas such as Celestial Seasonings, Red Zinger and Mandarin Orange, or Yogi Bhajan Teas. Red Bush (or Rooibosch) tea is good with milk and has a taste closer to 'normal' tea.

- **Chocolate** contains both sugar and chocolate. Start by having chocolate-free snacks, like Carriba bars. Then switch to chocolate- and sugar-free snacks such as cereal, fruit and nut bars. Then avoid even these, keeping them strictly for emergencies, eating fresh fruit instead if you feel you need something sweet.

- **Alcohol** is an easy habit to acquire because of its key role in social interaction. Start by limiting the times when you have alcohol. For example, don't drink at lunchtime. You'll certainly work better in the afternoon. Limit what you drink – for example, stick to wine, avoiding beer or spirits. Limit how much you drink by setting yourself a weekly target – for example, 7 glasses of wine a week. This allows you to have quite a few at that party on Saturday night and compensate by having little throughout the following week.

- **Smoking** can be one of the hardest habits to kick. The average smoker is not only addicted to nicotine, but is also addicted to smoking when tired, when hungry, when upset, on waking, after a meal, with a drink and so on. Improved nutrition decreases the craving for cigarettes. See the following pages for full details on how to give up.

How to Quit Smoking

One of the hardest stimulants to quit is cigarettes. Cigarettes contain nicotine, as well as 16 other cancer-producing chemicals. Nicotine, the primary stimulant, is more addictive than heroin and it produces a substantial effect even in small doses. In large amounts, it acts as a sedative. This is the attraction of nicotine: on the one hand it can give you a lift, on the other it can calm you down. Before a meal it can stop you feeling hungry and after a meal it can stop you feeling drowsy.

All these effects are due to nicotine's action on adrenal hormones, blood sugar and brain chemicals. By strictly following the advice given this week, your craving for cigarettes will diminish as a direct consequence of stabilising your blood sugar and hormone levels.

Ideally you quit cigarettes as you start your 6 Weeks to Superhealth programme. If you are trying to quit smoking at some other time, I recommend following the guidelines given here strictly for 2 months, preferably with the guidance and support of a clinical nutritionist, until you no longer consume any other stimulants (such as tea, coffee and chocolate) or sugar, instead eating small, frequent meals with an emphasis on foods containing slow-releasing carbohydrates combined with protein-rich foods. While it would be perfect to give up right now, the guidelines below are given for a 2-month quitting programme.

■ **Breaking the associated habits** If you are a smoker you are not only addicted to nicotine, but are also addicted to smoking at certain times – when you are tired, hungry or upset, on waking, after a meal, with a drink and so on. Before you actually give up smoking altogether it is best to break these mental associations.

Without attempting to change your smoking habits, keep a diary for a week (see page 52). Write down every situation in which you smoke. Describe how you feel before and how you feel after smoking.

When the week is up add up how many cigarettes you smoke associated with each situation. Your list might look something like this:

With a hot drink – 16	Difficult situation – 4
After a meal – 6	After sex – 3
With alcohol – 4	

Now set yourself targets. For the first week (or two) smoke as much as you like whenever you like but not when you drink a hot drink. For the next week (or two) smoke as much as you like whenever you like but not when

Day _____		
Time Situation	Feeling Before	Feeling After
9am With coffee	Tired	Awake

Smoking diary

you drink a hot drink or within 30 minutes of finishing a meal. Continue like this until, when you smoke, all you do is smoke, without the associated habits.

This will be tremendously helpful for you when you quit. Most people start again because the phone rings with a problem, someone brings in a coffee, offers you a cigarette . . . before you know it you're smoking.

■ **Reducing your nicotine load** Now it's time to reduce your nicotine load gradually. Week by week, switch to a brand that contains less nicotine until what you smoke contains no more than 2mg per cigarette. Supplementing the recommended 1,000mg of vitamin C and 200mcg of chromium should help reduce your cravings. You may also want to have 50mg of niacin with each meal – you may experience a blushing sensation when first taking it. This is harmless and usually occurs 15–30 minutes after taking it, for about 15 minutes. The blushing is less likely to occur if you take niacin with a meal and will diminish and, in most cases, stop completely if you take 50mg three times a day.

Increasing the alkaline balance of the body helps reduce cravings: a way to achieve this is by eating a diet that is high in fruit, vegetables and seeds, in other words, the one recommended throughout your 6 Weeks to Superhealth programme.

Whenever you feel the need for nicotine, first eat an apple or pear. This will raise a low blood sugar level, which is often the factor that triggers such a craving.

Regular exercise also helps, so the *Psychocalisthenics* which accompany each week of the programme should be useful.

Now reduce the number of cigarettes until you are smoking no more than 5 cigarettes a day, each with a nicotine content of 2mg or less. If you wish, stop smoking and replace with nicotine gum as an intermediate step. Nicotine gum comes in two strengths – 4mg and 2mg.

You want to be down to a maximum of 10mg of nicotine a day before quitting, i.e. 5 pieces of 2mg nicotine gum, or 5 × 2mg nicotine cigarettes.

■ **Time to quit** It is now time to quit and it is best to give yourself all the support you can get. Make sure your friends and work colleagues know so they can support you, not trying to stress you out or over-reacting if you are not at your best. It's great to have a buddy you can talk to whenever you are craving nicotine. They can help you strengthen your resolve.

The withdrawal effects from nicotine are a direct effect of its action on your blood sugar, so again, the recommendations for this week are ideal.

Beating the Sugar Blues and Snack Attacks

At first you may find it difficult coming off stimulants and you may actually suffer from withdrawal symptoms. This is temporary and rarely happens for more than 3 days as your blood sugar begins to return to normal stability. Often you get what is known as the 'sugar blues', or other symptoms such as headaches, fatigue, feeling shaky, irritability, anger or aches and pains. It is possible to lessen the blow of these symptoms and give yourself a much smoother ride by following a few easy tips:

- If your symptoms are intense, eat 4 or 5 small meals a day which all contain protein such as fish, soya products, nuts, cottage cheese or yoghurt.

- Aways eat a good breakfast containing some protein foods, for example porridge with ground seeds and yoghurt. This will keep blood sugar levels steady throughout the day.

- Eat fruit when you feel like reaching out for the wrong kind of snack or a stimulant. Have something exotic like kiwi, mango and passion fruit, or nibble on berries. Carry fruit with you when you go out in case of blood sugar drops. The best fruits for stabilising blood sugar are apples and pears. Have a few almonds too – the combination of slow-releasing sugars and protein in the almonds is excellent for stabilising blood sugar levels and hence energy.

- Remember that sugar is an acquired taste. So as you cut down the level of sweetness in *all* the food you eat you will soon get accustomed to this. When you want something sweet have fruit. Sweeten cereals and desserts with fruit. Let your taste buds be the judge of how sweet a food is – but do check the labels for all those disguised forms of sugar. You can always find a selection of sugar-free treats and biscuits in the health store, but save these for special occasions as you want to break the habit and cravings for sweet foods.

Watching your carbohydrate intake and reducing stress and stimulants now needs backing up by a third factor: nutrients.

3 Introduce Energy Nutrients

If you're thinking that all you need to do is eat complex carbohydrates and keep breathing, that's only half the story. Nutritional supplements are vital. All the chemical reactions which create energy are carefully controlled by enzymes, themselves dependent on no less than 8 vitamins and 5 minerals. Any shortage of these critical catalysts and your energy factories, the mitochondria, go out of tune. The result is inefficient energy production, a loss of stamina, highs and lows – or even just lows.

The minerals iron, calcium, magnesium, chromium and zinc are also vital for making energy. Calcium and magnesium are perhaps the most important, because all muscle cells need an adequate supply of these to be able to contract and relax. A shortage of magnesium, so common in people who don't eat much fruit or vegetables, often results in cramps, as muscles are unable to relax.

The older you are the less likely you are to be taking in enough chromium – an essential mineral that helps stabilise blood sugar levels. The average daily intake is below 50mcg, while an optimal intake, certainly for those with blood sugar problems, is around 200mcg. Chromium is found in wholefoods and is therefore higher in wholewheat flour, bread or pasta than in refined products, as well as in beans, nuts and seeds. Asparagus and mushrooms are especially rich in chromium. Since it works with insulin to help stabilise your blood sugar level, the more uneven your blood sugar level the more chromium you use up. Hence, a sugar and stimulant addict, eating refined foods, is most at risk of deficiency. Flour has 98 per cent of its chromium removed in the refining process – another reason to stay away from refined foods.

Nutritional supplements, taken on a regular basis, make a big difference to your overall experience of energy. The better you feel the more able you are to deal with stress. Also, the more stressful your life the more nutrients you need. Below are some of the most important nutrients needed to make energy:

B1 (thiamine)	25–100mg	Co-enzyme Q10	10–90mg
B2 (riboflavin)	25–100mg	Vitamin C	1,000–3,000mg
B3 (niacin)	50–150mg	Calcium	150–500mg
B5 (pantothenic acid)	50–200mg	Magnesium	100–3,000mg
B6 (pyridoxine)	50–100mg	Iron	5–15mg
B12(cyanocobalamin)	10–100mcg	Zinc	10–20mg
Folic acid	100–400mcg	Chromium	100–300mcg

Combine these supplements with the carbohydrate and stress-reducing suggestions for a healthier lifestyle.

ENERGY **Action Plan**

DOs

- Combine carbohydrate-rich foods with high-protein foods such as animal products, soy products or nuts.

- Eat 3 meals a day with 2 healthy snacks, rather than only having 1 or 2 large meals.

- Eat foods rich in B vitamins (wheatgerm, fish, green vegetables, wholegrains, mushrooms, eggs, etc.) and vitamin C (peppers, watercress, cabbage, broccoli, cauliflower, strawberries, lemons, kiwi fruit, oranges, tomatoes, etc.).

- Eat foods rich in magnesium (wheatgerm, almonds, cashew nuts, buckwheat, green vegetables), calcium (cheese, almonds, green vegetables, seeds, prunes, etc.), zinc (oysters, lamb, nuts, fish, egg yolk, wholegrains, almonds, etc.) and iron (pumpkin seeds, almonds, cashew nuts, raisins, pork, etc.).

And as always . . .

1 heaped tablespoon of ground seeds or 1 tablespoon of cold-pressed seed oil.

2 servings of beans, lentils, quinoa, tofu (soya), or 'seed' vegetables.

3 pieces of fresh fruit such as apples, pears, bananas, berries, melon or citrus fruit.

4 servings of wholegrains such as rice, millet, rye, oats, corn or quinoa.

5 servings of dark green, leafy and root vegetables such as watercress, carrots, sweet potatoes, broccoli, spinach, green beans, peas and peppers.

6 glasses of water, diluted juices, herb or fruit teas.

7 Eat whole, organic, raw food as much as you can.

8 Avoid any form of sugar, white, refined or processed food with chemical additives.

9 Avoid all stimulants – coffee, tea, cigarettes.

10 Relax during your meal and chew your food well.

DON'Ts

■ Avoid all stimulants – tea, coffee, cigarettes, chocolate, caffeinated drinks.

■ Avoid refined sugars, including honey.

■ Avoid refined carbohydrates, including white bread, biscuits, cakes, white rice and other processed foods.

■ Avoid alcohol.

■ Never skip breakfast.

■ Don't substitute sugar with sugar substitutes. These may not raise your blood sugar levels, but neither do they allow you to change your habits.

ENERGY-BOOSTING Menus

The emphasis here is based on providing a diet that both maintains sufficient blood sugar levels for consistent energy and avoids peaks and troughs in blood sugar levels which stimulate the release of stress-related hormones. Look at pages 54–6 for the basic advice on what to eat for energy. You can be as adventurous as you like. Here are some suggestions for daily menus designed to give you energy.

Breakfast

(Replace dairy foods with soya milk and yoghurt or rice milk.)
Choose from:
• Ultimate Power Breakfast (page 174)
• Get Up & Go (page 213) blended with skimmed or soya milk and a banana
• Millet or Rice Flake Porridge (page 177)
• Berry Booster (page 175)

Other recipes can be taken from *The Optimum Nutrition Cookbook* (Piatkus, 1999), which I co-authored with Judy Ridgway.

Lunch

Choose from:

- Spicy Lentil and Watercress Soup (page 187)
- Jacket Baked Potatoes with Tofu Topping (page 206)
- Lemon Chicken on Leafy Asparagus Salad (page 183)

Other recommended recipes, taken from the *The Optimum Nutrition Cookbook*, include: Provençal Vegetables with Goat's Cheese Dressing; Smoked Haddock Kedgeree with Grilled Tomatoes; Grilled Scallops on Green Leaves with Grated Celeriac; Ginger, Chicken and Beansprout Soup.

Dinner

Choose from:

- Grilled Scallops with Green Sauce, Julienne Vegetables and Rice Noodles (page 197)
- Pot Roasted Guinea Fowl with Spicy Potatoes and Wild Mushrooms in Sesame Sauce (page 204)
- Minted Trout with Grapefruit Rice Salad (page 199)

Other recommended recipes, taken from the *The Optimum Nutrition Cookbook*, include: Warm Avocado, Arame, Rice and Quinoa Salad with Rainbow Roots; Duck Slivers with Orange, Beansprouts and Chinese Egg Noodles; Mexican Spinach with Baked Yams; Grilled Carrot and Tofu Cakes with Red Peppers and Fennel.

ENERGY-BOOSTING Supplements

This week I recommend you take...

	Breakfast	Lunch	Dinner
Multi-vitamin/mineral	2		
Vitamin C 1,000mg	1		
Chromium 200mcg	1		

bananas   peaches/nectarines

kiwis   plums

mangos   figs

berries   (dried fruit)

pears

low fat, organic, natural yoghurt

5 seed mix - flax, sesame, pumpkin,
        sunflower & hemp.

wheatgerm

honey

nutmeg/vanilla essence.

skimmed milk

flaked rice/millet

Baking potatoes

ed to
acity.
acity,
ing is
itions
body.
own
, our
t ease
link
body.
y. By
ulate

h the
d the
rtless.
lying
uring

ne rib
body's
vidths
your

s you
point.
xhale,
m top

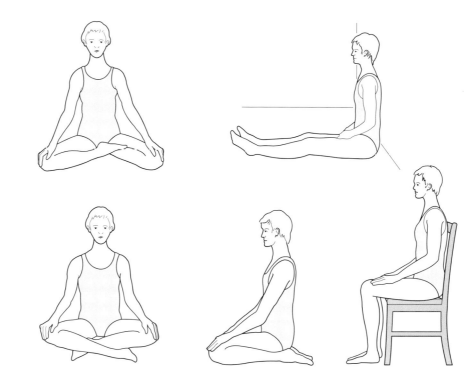

Dia-Kath breathing positions

1. Sit comfortably, in a quiet place with your spine straight in any one of the above positions.

2. Focus your attention in your *Kath* point.

3. Let your belly expand from the *Kath* point as you inhale slowly, deeply and effortlessly. Feel your diaphragm being pulled down towards the *Kath* point as your lungs fill with air from the bottom to the top.

On the exhale, relax both your belly and your diaphragm, emptying your lungs from top to bottom.

4. Repeat at your own pace.

- **Every morning sit down in a quiet place** before breakfast and practise Dia-Kath breathing for 5 minutes, or 36 breaths.

- **Whenever you are stressed throughout the day check your breathing.** Practise Dia-Kath breathing for 9 breaths. Dia-Kath breathing is great to do before an important meeting, or when something has upset you.

WEEK 1 Psychocalisthenics Exercises

On the following pages you will find the instructions for the first 4 exercises. Once you have perfected them, follow the complete routine for Week 1 which is set out on page 64.

Integration Breath

Foot position 2 foot-widths

Breathing *Inhale*, to a count of 6: *Exhale*, to a count of 6: Fill the lungs from the bottom to the top, breathing deeply with your concentration in the *Kath* or balance point. Empty your lungs from the top to the bottom.

Repeat ×3 at the beginning of your routine, and again ×1 after each of the other exercises (see pages 30 and 64). It should be repeated ×3 after Completo (see page 162).

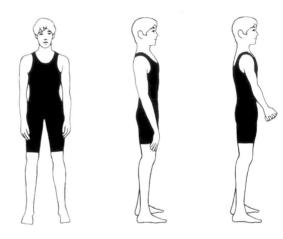

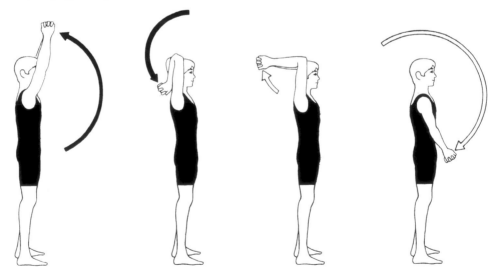

Points to note The outside edges of your feet are parallel. Your feet appear slightly pigeon-toed. Keep your knees unlocked and relaxed and your chin tucked in slightly. The imagery is of letting your hands float up behind the neck, pressing the palms together, and then letting your hands float back down. Count to 6 on the exhalation as well as on the inhalation.

Picking Grapes

Foot position 2 foot-widths

Breathing *Exhale*, swing down,
2 counts: *Inhale*, 4 pumps,
4 counts + 4 reaches, 4 counts

Repeat ×6

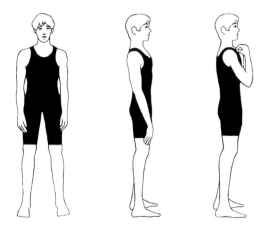

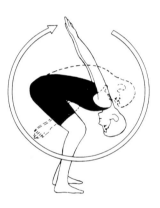

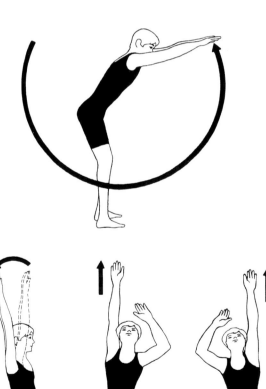

Points to note The knees bend during
the swing down. Swinging up, keep the
knees unlocked and relaxed, legs steady.
The 'pumps' of your shoulders and arms
lift the entire rib cage up and away from
the pelvis, as the rib cage is expanded by
the 4 quick inhalations. Feel the stretch
in your diaphragm area and in the upper
part of your abdominal muscles. Avoid
swaying the pelvis back and forth during
the 'pumping' motion. Stretch all the way
to your fingertips when 'picking', with 4
more quick inhalations.

Lateral Stretch

Foot position 3 foot-widths

Breathing *Inhale*, stretch left, 2 counts: *Exhale*, tuck, 1 count:
Inhale, stretch right, 2 counts: *Exhale*, tuck, 1 count

Repeat ×6

Points to note Move in a vertical plane as you stretch to each side – avoid
twisting the body. Feel the stretch from the crest of your hip bone, through
your waist, the sides of your rib cage, the armpit area, and along your arm into
your hand. The stretch curves directly over you. Look straight to the front.

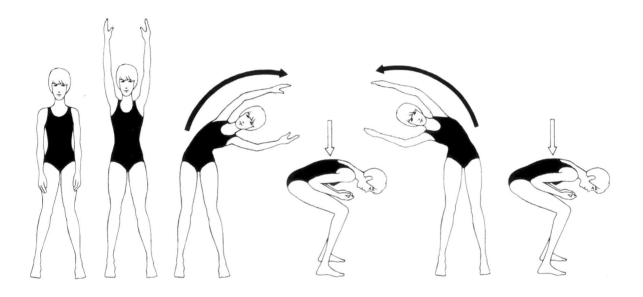

Flamingo

Foot position 1½ foot-widths

Breathing *Inhale*, drop over and rest, 3 counts: *Exhale*, up, 3 counts

Repeat ×6

Points to note Bending over, reach out 30 cm in front of your toes with your knuckles, stretching the muscles in the backs of your legs. Your weight transfers to the front of your feet. Feel the stretch through your hips and into the back. Come up keeping your back straight. Bending over, drop your head completely, looking back between your legs.

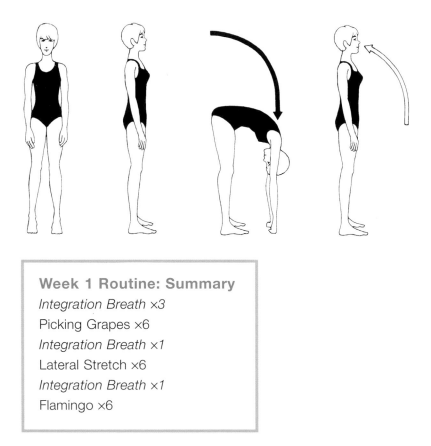

Week 1 Routine: Summary

Integration Breath ×3
Picking Grapes ×6
Integration Breath ×1
Lateral Stretch ×6
Integration Breath ×1
Flamingo ×6

You've reached the end of Week 1 of your 6 Weeks to Superhealth programme and you should already be feeling more alert and full of energy. Remember everything you've learnt as you move on to Week 2.

TUNE UP YOUR DIGESTION

Week 1 has been all about lowering our sugar, stress and stimulant levels. Now we're into Week 2, and ready to talk about the food we eat.

You Are Not What You Eat

You are not what you eat – you are what you can digest and absorb. Nothing is more important to your overall health than the health of your digestive tract. It is the interface between your body and the outside world. Over a lifetime no less than 100 tons of food passes along the digestive tract, much of it destined to become you. The digestive tract is your 'inside skin' and has a surface area the size of a small football pitch. Amazingly, most of the billions of cells that make up this barrier between your body and the environment are renewed every 4 days.

The digestive tract is the gateway into the body, jealously guarded by an immune army of bouncers, kept glorious and healthy by a careful balance of millions of health-promoting bacteria. Before food is ready to be presented to the inner kingdom of the body it must be prepared, broken down, digested. Only then is it invited as a guest to enter the body.

The fundamental design of the human body is a doughnut with a hole in the middle. The digestive tract represents the hole in the middle and is carefully designed to allow large food particles to be broken down into smaller units, capable of absorption into the body. The digestive tract, technically known as the gastrointestinal tract, is around 30 feet long and has various organs attached to it which produce digestive juices.

Problems of Digestion

The consequences of sub-optimum nutrition and unconscious eating are evident in the increasing incidence of digestive problems and the pattern of today's common diseases. There is no doubt that most of us are digging our own graves with a knife and fork. No longer is most of society's suffering the direct result of poverty. Indeed, much of the Western world's illness is the consequence of too much food, rather than too little, and of eating the wrong kinds of foods.

As a result, there is a quiet epidemic of digestive problems which include indigestion, irritable bowel syndrome, stomach bugs, ulcers, Crohn's, colitis and diverticulitis, candidiasis and chronic fatigue.

In 1933, Dr Anthony Bassler wrote after a 25-year study of over 5,000 cases, 'Every physician should realise that the intestinal toxaemias are the most important primary and contributing causes of many disorders and diseases of the human body.' Intestinal toxaemia, or toxicity, is not a condition that has disappeared – on the contrary, it is very much on the increase.

Whether or not you are currently suffering from any digestive problems, the chances are that you could tune up your digestion and reap the rewards in terms of extra health and energy. Week 2 is designed to help you do just that, by focusing on vital aspects of digestion: fibre, bacteria, wheat allergy and enzymes. The week ends with a detoxifying digestive spring-clean.

The Fibre Factor

We owe a lot to Drs Denis Burkitt and Hubert Trowell, who painstakingly travelled the world collecting stool samples! The conclusion of their research was that communities with loose-formed stools had very low incidence of colitis, diverticulitis, appendicitis, haemorrhoids and constipation, while communities with hardened, compacted stools were plagued by such digestive diseases as well as by the classic Western diseases of diabetes, heart disease and cancer. They identified the health-promoting factor as 'fibre'.

Not all types of carbohydrate can be digested and broken down into glucose. Indigestible carbohydrate is called fibre. Fibre is a natural constituent of a healthy diet that is high in fruits, vegetables, lentils, beans and wholegrains; by eating such a diet you have less risk of bowel cancer, diabetes or diverticular disease, and are unlikely to suffer from constipation.

Contrary to the popular image of fibre as mere 'roughage', it can actually absorb water and as it does so it makes faecal matter bulkier, less dense and easier to pass along the digestive tract. This decreases the amount of time food waste spends inside the body and reduces the risk of infection or cell changes due to carcinogens that are produced when some foods, particularly meat, degrade. The bulkier faecal matter also means less chance of a blockage, or constipation.

There are many different kinds of fibre, some of which are proteins, not carbohydrates. Some fibre, such as that found in oats, is called 'soluble fibre' and combines with sugar molecules to slow down the absorption of carbohydrates. It therefore helps to keep blood sugar levels balanced. Some fibre is much more water-absorbent than others. While wheat fibre swells to 10 times its original volume in water, glucomannan fibre, from the Japanese konjac plant, swells to 100 times its volume. Highly absorbent types of fibre, by bulking up foods and 'slow-releasing' sugars, can help to control appetite and play a part in weight maintenance.

The average daily intake of fibre in the UK and US is around 20 grams – less than half that of rural Africans, who consume around 55 grams a day and suffer from few of the lower digestive diseases so common in the West. An ideal intake of fibre is not less than 35 grams a day.

Provided the right foods are eaten (beans, lentils, peas or a large selection of crunchy vegetables, for example), 35 grams can easily be achieved without the need to add extra fibre. John Dickerson, Professor of Nutrition at the University of Surrey, has stressed the danger of adding wheat bran to a nutrient-poor diet. The reason for this is that wheat bran contains high levels of phytate, which reduces the absorption of essential minerals, including zinc. Overall, it is probably best to get a mixture of fibres from oats, lentils, beans, seeds, fruits and raw or lightly cooked vegetables. Much of the fibre in vegetables is destroyed by cooking, so vegetables are best eaten crunchy.

Week 2

CHECK YOUR DIGESTION

Complete this questionnaire to discover whether your digestive processes could be under par.

                                                                    C T

- Do you chew your food thoroughly?   Y Y
- Do you sometimes suffer from bad breath?   N N
- Do you often get a burning sensation in your stomach?   N N
- Do you often have a feeling of fullness in your stomach?   Y N
- Do you find it difficult digesting fatty foods?   N N
- Do you regularly use indigestion tablets?   Y N
- Do you get intermittent or ongoing diarrhoea?   Y N
- Do you get intermittent or ongoing constipation?   N N
- Do you often get a bloated stomach?   Y N
- Do you often belch or pass wind?   Y Y
- Do you often get stomach pains?   Y N
- Do you often feel nauseous?   N N
- Do you experience anal irritation?   N N
- Do you have a bowel movement less than once a day?   N N
- Do your stools rarely float?   Y N

- If you answer 'yes' to 7 or more questions there's a very good chance that your digestion needs support from changing your diet and supplements.

- If you answer 'yes' to between 4 and 7 questions you are beginning to show signs of digestive difficulties.

- If you answer 'yes' to fewer than 4 questions, you are unlikely to have a digestive problem, unless you suffer severely from only a couple of the symptoms.

Promoting Healthy Intestinal Flora

Did you know that up to 4lb (1.8kg) of your body weight comes from bacteria? The average person has around 400 different types of friendly bacteria, mainly resident in the digestive tract, which are forever multiplying. There are about 100 trillion bacteria in your digestive tract, most of which are in the colon. That's more than the total number of cells in your body. Every day you make several ounces of bacteria and eliminate an equal amount in stools.

Not all of these bacteria are good for you, but provided you have enough of the health-promoting ones, they act as the first line of defence against unfriendly bacteria and other disease-producing microbes including viruses and fungi. The good ones also make some vitamins and digest fibre, allowing us to derive more nutrients from otherwise indigestible food, and also help promote a healthy digestive environment.

Probiotics

So the right kind of bacteria are our friends, and are known as 'intestinal flora' or probiotics. The principle friendly bacteria include the families of *Lactobacillus* and *Bifidus* bacteria. The *Bifidus* family of bacteria generally make up a quarter of the total flora in the digestive tract. Taking supplements of these friendly bacteria gives pathogenic (harmful) bacteria less chance of survival. There are many different strains of friendly bacteria, some of which actually live in the gut, while others simply 'pass through' and are useful while they're there. Here are the principal friendly bacteria:

	Children	**Adults**
Resident	B. infantis	L. acidophilus
	B. bifidum	B. bacterium
		L. salivarius
		Enterococci
Passing through	L. bulgaricus	L. casei (from cheese)
	S. thermophilus	S. thermophilus
		L. salivarius
		L. bulgaricus

Key: B = *Bifidobacteria*   L = *Lactobacillus*   S = *Streptococcus*

Those that are resident, sometimes called 'human strain', are usually more powerful at fighting infection because they multiply and colonise the digestive tract. Others are available in fermented foods such as yoghurt, miso and sauerkraut. Yoghurt and other fermented dairy products often contain *Lactobacillus thermophilus* or *L. bulgaricus*. These bacteria will hang around for a week or so doing good work. They, like the other beneficial bacteria, can make vitamins as well as turning lactose, the main sugar in milk, into lactic acid. This makes the digestive tract slightly more acidic, which inhibits disease-causing microbes such as *Candida albicans* from multiplying. Overall, eating a plant-based diet, high in fruits and vegetables, which are naturally high in fibre, is much more likely to encourage healthy bacteria.

The benefits of having a healthy population of beneficial bacteria are many:

- **They make vitamins** including vitamins B1, B2, B3, B5, B6, B12, biotin, A and K.

- **They fight infections** and have been shown to halve recovery time from diarrhoea, prevent overgrowth of salmonella and *E.coli*, the bacteria responsible for many cases of food poisoning, *Helicobacter pylori* and *Candida albicans*.

- **They boost immunity** by increasing the number of immune cells.

- **They promote other 'good' bacteria while reducing 'bad' bacteria** *Lactobacillus acidophilus* supplementation, for instance, has been shown to promote the beneficial *Bifidobacteria* and inhibit disease-producing microbes.

- **They repair and promote health of the digestive tract** because beneficial bacteria ferment sugars into short-chain fatty acids such as butyric acid, which is used as fuel by the intestinal lining, helping it to repair.

- **They are anti-inflammatory** and have been shown to help conditions such as arthritis.

- **They are anti-allergy** and have been shown to help reduce inflammatory reactions in food allergies by lessening the response in the gut to allergenic foods.

Many food reactions may be due not solely to food allergy but also to the feeding of unfriendly bacteria which then produce substances that activate the immune system in the gut.

Reinoculate Your Digestive Tract with Probiotics

If you have had a major infection or have been treated with antibiotics, you may benefit from a more direct way of 'reinoculating' your digestive tract by taking a probiotic supplement. The more 'broad-spectrum' the antibiotic the more likely it is to devastate your colony of beneficial bacteria, leaving you even more susceptible to infection. Actually, most of us could do with a boost of these friendly bugs anyway.

Healthfood stores stock probiotic supplements, many of which contain a combination of beneficial bacteria. The two most common families of bacteria provided are *Lactobacillus acidophilus* and the *Bifidobacteria*. Different strains are included for supplements designed for children or adults, so it's wise to seek advice on the best one to take, depending on your circumstances.

Our Deadly Bread

One of the most common intestinal irritants is wheat. Wheat is rich in a protein called gluten that contains gliadin, which is known to irritate the intestines. A small amount may be tolerated, but many people consume wheat in the form of biscuits, toast, bread, cereals, cakes, pastry and pasta at least 3 times a day.

Modern wheat is much richer in gluten and hence in gliadin. This is because gluten, while bad news for your digestion, is good news for the baking industry. When yeast is fed sugar it produces gas. In the presence of the sticky protein gluten this makes bubbles, and hence lighter loaves. This makes baked products look bigger and sell better. This kind of baking increases the amount of gluten which has the potential to react with the gut wall.

While a high gluten diet is bad news for anyone, as this sticky protein can gunk up and irritate the digestive tract, some people are more severely sensitive to it. They have what is called coeliac disease, in which the tiny protrusions that make up the small intestine – the villi – get worn away, which results in all sorts of symptoms and malabsorption problems and a consequent loss of weight.

Digestive Problems and Wheat

A study at the Institute for Optimum Nutrition investigated the effects of removing wheat from the diet of 66 people who had digestive problems. They all craved bread, and as a result ate a lot of it; none of them knew that wheat might be causing the digestive problems. They abstained from eating wheat for a period of 6 weeks to investigate the possibility of food allergy or intolerance.

Results showed that 90 per cent of the participants had improvements in all of their digestive symptoms. Of these, 6 per cent had between 75 and 100 per cent improvement in all their symptoms. Dramatic reduction was shown in 6 symptoms: constipation, flatulence, bloating, food cravings, lack of energy and mood swings. It is reasonable to suggest that these subjects were suffering from wheat intolerance.

The most common symptoms of wheat sensitivity are constipation, diarrhoea, abdominal bloating or pain. However, many other symptoms have also been reported in those found to be sensitive to wheat.

WHEAT CHECK

How much wheat do you eat each day?   **portions per day**

bread	☐	☐	☐	☐	☐	☐	☐	☐	☐
cereals	☐	☐	☐	☐	☐	☐	☐	☐	☐
biscuits	☐	☐	☐	☐	☐	☐	☐	☐	☐
cake slices	☐	☐	☐	☐	☐	☐	☐	☐	☐
pasta	☐	☐	☐	☐	☐	☐	☐	☐	☐

Tick a box for every portion eaten   **Total** ☐

Are you sensitive to wheat?

Do you suffer from . . .	fatigue	anxiety and paranoia	throat troubles
nausea	sweating	cramps	skin rashes
abdominal bloating	acne and boils	flatulence	migraine
constipation	apathy and confusion	diarrhoea	depression

If you suffer from any of the above symptoms and are eating 3 servings of wheat or more a day, you may well be sensitive to wheat. You may find that continuing to avoid it, or eating it only once every 4 days, helps, after it has been reintroduced into your diet during your 6 Weeks to Superhealth programme.

If you are eating more than 7 servings of wheat a day, I strongly recommend that you aim to reduce this, even after wheat is reintroduced into your diet.

Often, as part of a digestive healing programme, it is wise to go on a no-wheat diet for a month. Fortunately, there are many wheat-free options to choose from in healthfood shops and supermarkets these days.

- **Breads** Rye bread, corn bread, rice cakes, oat cakes.

- **Pasta** Buckwheat spaghetti, soba noodles (buckwheat), rice noodles, quinoa pasta, corn pasta.

- **Cereals** Cornflakes, oatmeal, rice cereal, millet flakes and other types available at healthfood stores.

- **Other starchy foods** Sweet potato, brown rice, potato, polenta (maize).

Enzymes – the Keys of Life

The food we eat is made out of large, complex molecules that couldn't possibly enter into the body. First they have to be broken down into much smaller particles which not only are physically able to get through the wall of the digestive tract but are also 'on the guest list'. This breaking down is the job of digestive enzymes.

These enzymes are produced in large amounts at different stages along the digestive tract. If you don't produce enough of them to digest your food, you can end up with immediate indigestion, bloating and flatulence. The long-term effects of having undigested food in your system, however, are more insidious and can lead to a greater risk for inflammatory bowel syndrome and digestive infections such as candidiasis and allergies.

Carbohydrate digestion begins in the mouth through the action of the enzyme ptyalin. Ptyalin is an 'amylase', which is the name given to enzymes that digest carbohydrate. Carbohydrate doesn't get further digested in the stomach, so it theoretically passes straight into the duodenum, where amylase enzymes that pour into the duodenum – out of the pancreatic duct and cells that line the upper part of the small intestine – further break down carbohydrate.

In contrast to carbohydrate, protein is digested principally in the stomach. For this reason the stomach produces two substances: hydrochloric acid and an enzyme called pepsinogen. Hydrochloric acid, commonly called stomach acid, gets to work on the big protein molecules straight away, but its action alone is limited. When the body combines pepsinogen and hydrochloric acid, however, a very powerful enzyme called pepsin is created. This starts to break down complex proteins into relatively small chunks of amino acids, called peptides, which are further broken down into individual amino acids by more protein-digesting enzymes, collectively known as proteases, which are produced by the

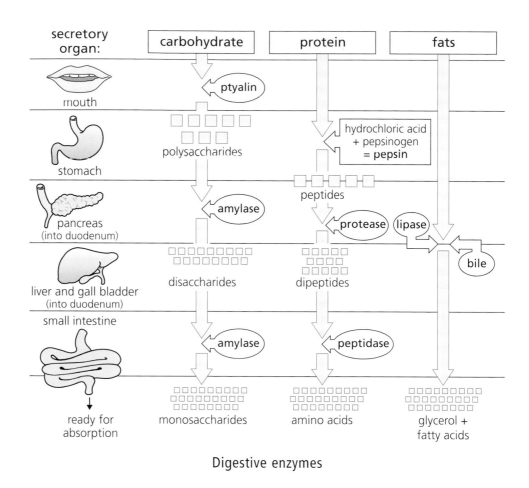

secretory organ:	carbohydrate	protein	fats
mouth	ptyalin		
stomach	polysaccharides	hydrochloric acid + pepsinogen = pepsin	
pancreas (into duodenum)	amylase	peptides protease	lipase
liver and gall bladder (into duodenum)	disaccharides	dipeptides	bile
small intestine			
	amylase	peptidase	
ready for absorption	monosaccharides	amino acids	glycerol + fatty acids

Digestive enzymes

pancreas and special cells in the first part of the small intestine. The end result, if all is going well, is that complex proteins end up as simple amino acids, ready for absorption.

Fat is a whole different story. While protein and carbohydrate are effectively water-soluble and can be acted on by the enzymes in digestive juices, fat repels water so these enzymes would have a very hard time getting a grip on fat. For this reason, the first stage of digesting fat, called emulsification, is all about actually preparing fat particles for digestion. This is done by a substance called bile, which is made in the liver and stored in the gall bladder. What bile does is break down large fat globules into tiny droplets of fat. The net consequence of effectively turning a football into 15 tennis balls is that there is a much greater surface area exposed to digestive juices. Once again, the pancreas plays a key role because the digestive juices it produces and sends into the duodenum contain lipase, a fat-digesting enzyme.

The Acid Test

Although not an enzyme, one of the most critical factors in digestion is stomach acid. Too much or too little is a common cause of digestive problems. Not only is stomach acid the prerequisite to all protein digestion, it is also necessary for mineral absorption and is the body's first line of defence against infections, effectively sterilising your food. So a lack of stomach acid (hydrochloric acid) leaves you unable to digest properly and prone to infections. This can lead to indigestion, particularly noticeable with high-protein meals, and the likelihood of developing food allergies because undigested large protein molecules are more likely to stimulate allergic reactions in the small intestine.

ARE YOU PRODUCING TOO LITTLE STOMACH ACID?

- Do you often get heartburn/indigestion?
- Do you often have a feeling of fullness or heaviness in your upper abdomen?
- Do you feel that food doesn't move along, it just 'sits there'?
- Do you feel hungrier after you have eaten?
- Do you often have a bloated belly and/or gas?
- Do you often get constipated?
- Can you often see undigested food in your stools?
- Is your tongue often coated?
- Do you suffer from bad breath?

If you answer 'yes' to more than 3 of the questions, you may well be producing too little stomach acid for good digestion, absorption and other functions. In which case, you could carry out the test described below.

You can do a test at home to give a rough indication of whether any burning in the stomach is due to excess or insufficient stomach acid. Please note, though, that in cases of persistent discomfort, more serious problems such as a stomach ulcer should first be ruled out by a doctor. The test involves taking a tablespoon of cider vinegar or lemon juice when you feel the acidity. If this helps the situation, it is possible that you are not producing enough stomach acid; if it makes it worse, then you may be producing too much. A health practitioner can advise you on what steps to take, either way.

Solving Indigestion

One of the main reasons for indigestion is that a person doesn't produce enough of all these enzymes to digest food properly. This means that incompletely digested food hangs around in the small intestine feeding the bacteria that live there. These bacteria produce gas, resulting in bloating, flatulence and digestive pain. Stomach acid release can also be a problem.

The first action to take if you've got indigestion is to supplement digestive enzymes, the main three being amylase, protease and lipase. Make sure you get one that contains all of these and take one with each meal.

Another way to restore the health of your digestive system is to give it a 'spring-clean', by following a detoxification schedule.

Digestive Spring-clean

We have all become more and more aware of the increasing pollution in our environment, in our water and food, and of the poisons and micro-organisms in our bodies that can lead to disease. Although the human body appears to be a vulnerable and sensitive organism, we have in fact been built to survive in an ocean of toxicity, and we have a number of ways of excluding, detoxifying and eliminating poisons. Only by understanding clearly how we build up toxicity can we reverse the process through cleansing and detoxification.

What Can You Do to Help?

The Western diet has been shown repeatedly to be lacking in vitality and freshness, to be low in fibre and too refined. Industrial food production has led to low levels of vitamins and minerals and high quantities of preservatives and other additives. Meat consumption can raise the putrefactive bacteria, while milk can increase the less desirable *Streptococcus* species of bacteria. Vegetables, on the other hand, promote the beneficial *Lactobacillus acidophilus* and *Bifidobacteria*. On average, vegetarians and organic food eaters are simply much healthier.

Colon-cleansing

Having said this, diet alone is neither the quickest nor the most effective way to restore digestive health. In addition to a diet that provides key nutrients and removes digestive irritants, certain herbs and fibres can help to cleanse the digestive tract and calm down inflammation. Combinations of these herbs and fibres are available in a number of 'colon-cleansing' powders and capsules. These are recommended as part of my programme for restoring digestive health. My favourite remedies are Higher Nature's Colo-Fibre and Colo-Clear (see Supplemental Options on page 213), based on the research of Brian Wright, author of *The Colon Health Handbook*.

One of the keys to good digestive health is making sure your food passes through you neither too slowly nor too quickly. If it goes through very slowly, food putrefies, feeding bad bacteria, producing gas, leaving toxins to be reabsorbed and irritating the gut lining, while a speedy passage means that there is not sufficient time for nutrients to be well absorbed, in effect leaving you malnourished.

Not all fibres are the same. Some, such as wheat bran, are quite irritating to the digestive tract and not ideal for restoring digestive health. Special herbal sources of fibre, when mixed with water, act as mucins, or gels, which both add bulk and are soothing because they help to calm down inflammation in the intestines. They also absorb toxic material and help to eliminate it. Brian Wright recommends the following combination of colon-cleansing fibres and herbs: linseed, psyllium husks, slippery elm, pectin, fennel, fenugreek, acacia gum, alfalfa, blessed thistle, cayenne, milk thistle, red clover. Organic golden flax seeds are another good intestinal cleanser – left to soak, they absorb water and become gel-like so that when they are eaten they cleanse the intestines and bulk out the stool.

Test Your Transit Time

To check your transit time – the length of time it takes for food to pass from one end of your digestive tract to the other – the easiest and most reliable test is simply to eat some beetroot or sweetcorn. Note the time that you eat it; then take a glance at what you pass each time you have a bowel movement.

	Time eaten and date	Time passed and date
Beetroot		
Sweetcorn		

The amount of time that it takes from when you eat the foods to when you see a dark red stool, or pieces of sweetcorn kernel, is your transit time. Ideally this should not be any longer than 24 hours. If your transit time is less than 12 hours you may not be absorbing all the nutrients from your food and are advised to investigate the possibility of allergies and malabsorption problems. If your transit time is more than 24 hours this indicates that waste material is spending too long inside you, a factor which increases your risk for colon-related diseases. This is a signal to increase your fibre intake and take some exercise which strengthens abdominal muscles.

Laboratory Tests

If you scored more than 8 in the main questionnaire on page 68, it may well be worth visiting a clinical nutritionist (see page 216), who can recommend which of the laboratory tests would be most useful to assess the health and function of your digestive tract. Stool tests can be done to check how well you are digesting and absorbing food, whether your gut contains sufficient friendly bacteria, any harmful organisms or an overgrowth of yeast. Other tests can be done to check stomach acid secretion and how well your stomach is emptying into the intestine.

DIGESTION-TUNING **Action Plan**

DOs

- Drink at least 1.5 litres of pure water throughout the day.

- Include in your diet plenty of foods which are naturally high in fibre, such as wholegrains, e.g. brown rice, oats, rye, barley, quinoa, buckwheat. Also root vegetables, lentils and beans.

- Eat live, natural, organic yoghurt (soya or dairy) daily.

- Soak a dessertspoon of organic golden linseeds in a glass of water overnight. Drink the mixture in the morning.

- Sit down, relax and take your time over your meals.

- Chew your food thoroughly.

And as always . . .

1 heaped tablespoon of ground seeds or 1 tablespoon of cold-pressed seed oil.

2 servings of beans, lentils, quinoa, tofu (soya), or 'seed' vegetables.

3 pieces of fresh fruit such as apples, pears, bananas, berries, melon or citrus fruit.

4 servings of wholegrains such as rice, millet, rye, oats, corn or quinoa.

5 servings of dark green, leafy and root vegetables such as watercress, carrots, sweet potatoes, broccoli, spinach, green beans, peas and peppers.

6 glasses of water, diluted juices, herb or fruit teas.

7 Eat whole, organic, raw food as much as you can.

8 Avoid any form of sugar, white, refined or processed food with chemical additives.

9 Avoid all stimulants − coffee, tea, cigarettes.

10 Relax during your meal and chew your food well.

DON'Ts

- Avoid all wheat – this includes bread, pasta, crackers, biscuits, cakes, pastry, most breakfast cereals, pizza and anything that contains flour including many sauces and batters. See page 73 for alternatives.

- Avoid all red meat. Use fish, soya products, lean chicken and some dairy products such as cottage cheese as sources of protein.

- Don't eat on the move or standing up.

- Don't have several different types of food in one meal.

- Don't drink more than just a small glass of water with meals.

- Limit your alcohol intake to no more than 2 units on 2 nights of the week, ideally red wine.

Week 2

DIGESTION-TUNING **Menus**

Below are some meal recommendations for Week 2. You can of course use or adapt recipes from other weeks which comply to the current 'Dos and Don'ts'.

Breakfast
- Choose from:
- Ultimate Power Breakfast (page 174)
- Get Up & Go (page 213) blended with skimmed or soya milk and a banana
- Breakfast Omelettes (page 178)
- Anton Mosimann's Oat Muesli with Fruit (page 175)

Other recipes can be taken from *The Optimum Nutrition Cookbook* (Piatkus, 1999), which I co-authored with Judy Ridgway.

Lunch
- Choose from:
- Winter Salad Platter with Tangy Cucumber Dressing (page 179)
- Gazpacho (page 185)
- Chicken Salad with Horseradish Sauce (page 181)

Other recommended recipes, taken from *The Optimum Nutrition Cookbook*, include: Oriental Vegetables with Tofu; Beetroot and Smoked Herring Salad with Spinach and Fennel Salad; Avocado and Tofu Dip Sandwich; Green Root Soup.

Dinner
Choose from:
- Flash Grilled Tuna in Lemon Ginger Marinade with Quinoa and Red Pepper Salsa (page 196)
- Potato, Coriander and Courgette Pie (page 209)
- Garden Paella (page 200)

Other recommended recipes, taken from *The Optimum Nutrition Cookbook*, include: Sesame Grilled Chicken on Celeriac Mash with Green Beans; Lemon and Dill Turkey Escalopes on Carrot and Tarragon Potato Mash with Beetroot Relish; Baked Aubergines with Peppers, Quinoa and Broccoli Salsa.

DIGESTION-TUNING **Supplements**

As always	BREAKFAST	LUNCH	DINNER
Multi-vitamin/mineral	2		
Vitamin C 1,000mg	1		
Add			
Digestive enzymes	1	1	1
Optional			
Probiotics	1		1
Colofibre	2	2	2
Colocleanse	1	1	1
Herbal Aloe Detox	1 tablespoon		1 tablespoon

- Take probiotics if you have taken a course of antibiotics in the last year.
- Take Colo-Fibre and Colocleanse or Herbal Aloe Detox if your transit time (see page 77) was more than 24 hours and/or if you suffer from excessive bloating and flatulence.

Optional to continue	BREAKFAST	LUNCH	DINNER
Chromium 200mcg	1		

DIGESTION-TUNING **Awareness Exercise**

Mindful Eating

As simple as it may sound, the act of digesting and absorbing nutrients from food is a highly complex and carefully orchestrated affair. From the moment you think about food, then see it, smell it, taste it and chew it, the digestive tract is getting ready by preparing the right digestive juices to deal with the meal.

Every time you eat a meal:

- **Smell your food** before you eat it.

- **Think about its origin** and be thankful in the knowledge that these molecules of food will literally become you.

- **Chew each mouthful completely** before beginning the next.

- **Take some time out for your meals** and either eat alone or in good company.

Week 2

WEEK 2 **Psychocalisthenics Exercises**

Add the following 3 exercises, summarised on page 84, to the routine you learnt in Week 1.

Ax 1

Foot position 5 foot-widths

Breathing *Inhale*, swing up to the left, 2 counts: *Exhale*, swing down to the right and follow through, 2 counts: *Inhale*, swing up to the right, 2 counts: *Exhale*, swing down to the left and follow through, 2 counts

Repeat ×6

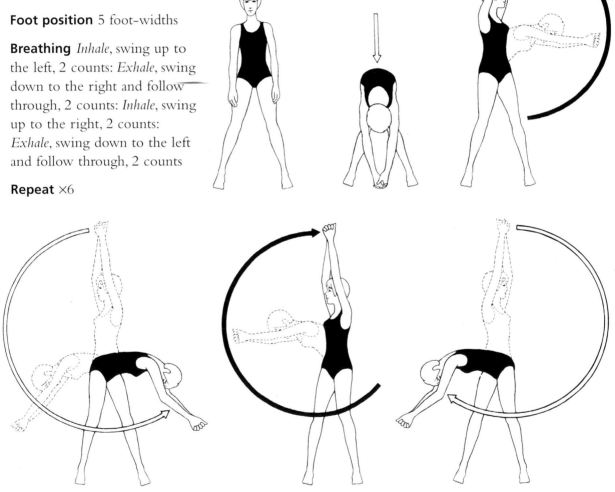

Points to note The inhale lasts through the full upswing, and the exhale starts at the beginning of the downswing and lasts all the way through. Let the breathing move the exercise. Extending your arms, rather than bending them at the elbows, stretches the lower back and abdominal muscles more.

Ax 2

Foot position 5 foot-widths

Breathing *Exhale*, 1 count: *Hold breath*, turn left, 1 count: *Inhale*, make 3 circles down to the left, up to the right, 6 counts (1 long breath): *Exhale*, 1 count: *Hold breath*, turn right, 1 count: *Inhale*, make 3 circles down to the right, up to the left, 6 counts (1 long breath)

Repeat ×3

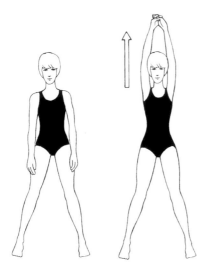
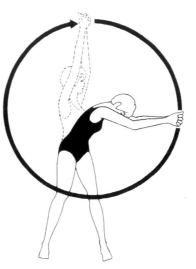

Points to note The correct breathing is one long continuous inhalation throughout the 3 circles, then a quick full exhalation at the top. To inhale evenly throughout the 3 circles, it is helpful to imagine your breath as a slender thread of air flowing continuously in your lungs, filling them from the bottom to the top. To keep your head between your arms as you make the rotations, it helps to imagine a connection between your ears and upper arms.

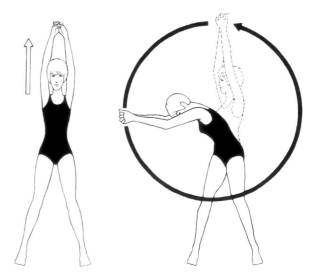

Udiyama

Foot position 3 foot-widths

Breathing *Inhale*, 3 counts: *Exhale*, 3 counts: *Hold breath*, contract and release muscles, 9 counts

Repeat ×3

Points to note To get the correct 45 degree inclination, bend your knees and tilt your torso and head forward, bringing your hands to rest lightly on your thighs. Your head and spine are in a straight line. Avoid bending over too far. The correct stance makes the contraction of the abdominal muscles massage the internal organs most effectively. You can feel the pull from the pubic bone up to the throat.

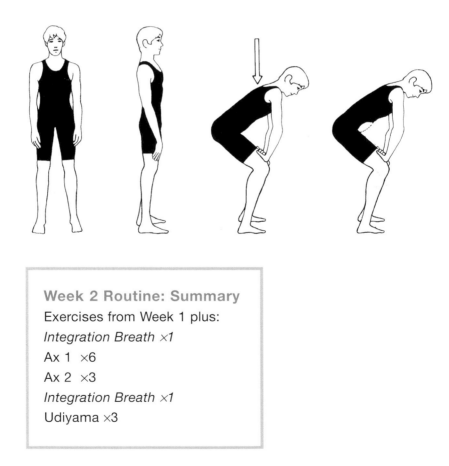

Week 2 Routine: Summary
Exercises from Week 1 plus:
Integration Breath ×1
Ax 1 ×6
Ax 2 ×3
Integration Breath ×1
Udiyama ×3

By following the regime in Week 2 of your 6 Weeks to Superhealth programme your digestion should now be well on the way towards recovery.

WEEK 3

BALANCE YOUR HORMONES

This week of 6 Weeks to Superhealth deals with your hormonal balance. Some of the most powerful chemicals in the body are hormones. They are produced in special glands which tell body cells what to do. Insulin, for example, tells the cells to take up glucose from the blood. Thyroxine, from the thyroid gland, speeds up the metabolism of cells, generating energy and burning fat. Oestrogen and progesterone, from the ovaries, control a sequence of changes that maintain fertility and the menstrual cycle. Hormone imbalances can wreak havoc with your health.

Hormones are made from components in food, so diet can play a crucial part in keeping their levels in balance. Most hormones work on feedback loops with the pituitary gland as the master of the orchestra. For example, the pituitary releases thyroid stimulating hormone (TSH), which tells the thyroid gland to release thyroxine which speeds up the metabolism of cells in the body. When the blood level of thyroxine reaches a certain point the pituitary stops producing TSH.

The Thyroid and Metabolism

The thyroid hormone thyroxine is made from the amino acid tyrosine, itself derived from the protein you eat. The enzyme that converts one into the other is dependent on iodine. A lack of either tyrosine or iodine can reduce thyroxine levels, although deficiency of either is quite rare. However, an underactive thyroid, which can be the cause of symptoms such as weight gain, mental and physical lethargy, constipation and thickening skin, is quite common. Many people suspected of thyroid problems have borderline 'normal' thyroxine levels on testing, but can have amazing health transformations from taking a low dose of thyroxine.

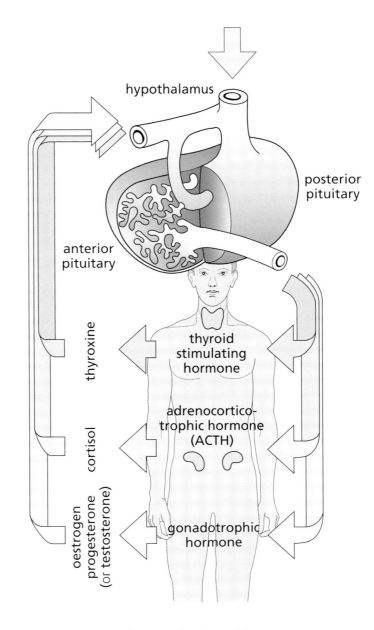

The endocrine glands and hormones

Maintaining Calcium Balance

The thyroid gland also produces a hormone responsible for maintaining calcium balance in the body. Calcitonin from the thyroid works in balance with parathormone (or PTH) from the parathyroid glands, four tiny glands attached to the thyroid. PTH converts vitamin D into an active hormone that helps to increase available calcium.

Stress and the Adrenals

The adrenal glands sit on top of the kidneys and produce hormones that, among other things, help us adapt to stress. The hormones adrenalin, cortisol and DHEA help us respond in an emergency by channelling the body's energy towards being able to 'fight or take flight', improving oxygen and glucose supply to muscles. The body slows down digestion, repair and maintenance to channel energy for dealing with stress. As a consequence, prolonged stress is associated with speeding up ageing and a number of diseases of digestion and hormone balance. More information on energy and stress is given in Week 1, page 38.

Sex Hormones

In women, the balance between progesterone and oestrogen is critical. A relative excess of oestrogen, called 'oestrogen dominance', is associated with an increased risk of breast cancer, fibroids, ovarian cysts, endometriosis and PMS. Common early warning symptoms of oestrogen dominance include PMS, depression, loss of sex drive, sweet cravings, heavy periods, weight gain, breast swelling and water retention.

Oestrogen dominance can occur due to excess exposure to oestrogenic substances, or a lack of progesterone, or a combination of both. Oestrogenic substances are found in meat, much of which is hormone-fed, dairy products, many herbicides and pesticides, and soft plastics, some of which leach into food when used for food wrapping. Oestrogen is also in most birth control pills and HRT.

If a woman doesn't ovulate, which is quite common after the age of 35, no progesterone is produced. This is because progesterone is produced in the sac that contains the ovum only if the ovum is released. Because of this, women are more likely to suffer from oestrogen dominance.

Week 3

Men, however, can also suffer from oestrogen dominance and testosterone deficiency. While men actually produce very little oestrogen, they are exposed to dietary and environmental sources of it. Some, such as the pesticide DDT, are known to interfere with the body's testosterone, creating a deficiency. This may explain the increase in the incidence of genital defects and undescended testes in male infants, as well as the rise in male infertility, impotency, prostate and testicular cancer. In later life some men have the equivalent of a 'male menopause'.

CHECK YOUR HORMONE BALANCE

Complete this questionnaire to discover whether your hormones may be out of balance.

Women

- Have you ever used or do you use the contraceptive pill? Y
- Have you had a hysterectomy or have you been sterilised? N
- Do you experience cyclical water retention? N
- Do you have excess hair on your body or thinning hair on your scalp? N
- Have you gained weight on your thighs and hips? Y
- Have you at any time been bothered with problems affecting your reproductive organs (ovaries or womb)? N
- Do you have fertility problems, difficulty conceiving or a history of miscarriage? N
- Are your periods often irregular or heavy? N
- Do you suffer from lumpy breasts? N
- Do you suffer from reduced libido or loss of interest in sex? N
- Do you often suffer from cyclical mood swings or depression? Y
- Do you suffer from insomnia? N
- Do you experience cramps or other menstrual irregularities? N
- Do you suffer from anxiety, panic attacks or nervousness? N
- Do you suffer from hot flushes or vaginal dryness? N

Men

- Have you had a vasectomy? ☑
- Are you gaining weight? ☑
- Do you often suffer from mood swings or depression? ☑
- Have you at any time been bothered with problems affecting your reproductive organs (prostate or testes)? ☑
- Do you suffer from reduced libido or loss of interest in sex? ☑
- Do you suffer from impotence? ☑
- Do you awake less frequently with a morning erection or have difficulty maintaining an erection? ☑
- Do you suffer from fatigue or loss of energy? ☑
- Do you suffer from anxiety or nervousness? ☑
- Do you suffer from irritability or anger? ☑
- Have you had a drop in your motivation and drive? ☑
- Do you feel that you are ageing prematurely? ☑
- Do you easily become stressed? ☑
- Do you have back problems or joint pains? ☑
- Do you have night sweats or suffer from excessive sweating? ☑

Week 3

- If you answer 'yes' to more than 7 questions, in either questionnaire, it is almost definite that you are suffering from a hormone imbalance.

- If you answer 'yes' to between 4 and 7 questions it is probable that hormone imbalance is a problem for you, so this needs to be improved.

- If you have answered 'yes' to less than 4 questions you are unlikely to have a hormone imbalance unless you have problems with libido, impotence, reduced potency or hot flushes.

- If you have had a vasectomy, a hysterectomy or a sterilisation then it is more likely that you have a hormone imbalance.

Two areas of life in which our hormones can get out of balance are menstruation and menopause. By following the guidelines, these can become less of a problem.

Beating PMS

Luckily for most women, premenstrual syndrome (PMS) is increasingly recognised as a real health problem. It comes in the form of any of a number of symptoms which occur only during the 2 weeks leading up to a period and are usually gone shortly after menstruation starts. Each woman will experience her unique combination of symptoms, and common ones include: anxiety, irritability, fluid retention, mood swings, bloating, breast tenderness, weight gain, acne, fatigue, sweet cravings, forgetfulness, headaches and depression.

The main categories of PMS are:

- **PMS associated with high oestrogen and low progesterone levels** Symptoms can be bloating, mood swings, fluid retention and breast tenderness. To reduce oestrogen levels it is useful to increase fibre, eat organically grown produce, limit exposure to hormone-disrupting compounds (see page 103 of this week's Awareness Exercise) and reduce consumption of high-fat meat and dairy produce.

- **PMS associated with food cravings** Eating nutritious wholefoods dense in nutrients and avoiding refined sugar should help control cravings. Magnesium, chromium and the essential fats (i.e. evening primrose or flax oils) are often deficient.

- **PMS associated with water retention** B6, magnesium and vitamin E have been shown to be helpful. Reducing sodium (salt) intake is also beneficial. Excess sodium increases the likelihood of developing water retention.

Other useful nutrients are magnesium, a deficiency of which is associated with poor appetite, nausea, apathy, tiredness, mood changes and muscle cramps. B vitamins are also important for the production of energy and stabilising mood.

It is entirely possible to become more or less symptom-free. Symptoms have been known to completely disappear in 90 per cent of women within 4 months of changing their diet, doing some exercise and finding effective ways of dealing with stress. There are very good supplements available that are especially blended to deal with the symptoms of PMS. Look out for products which contain the vitamins and minerals listed on the previous page and also herbs such as dong quai or white peony root. See page 99 for more information on what is available.

PMS CHECK

In the 2 weeks leading up to your period . . .

- Do you experience cramps or other menstrual irregularities?
- Do you easily become irritable or have angry outbursts?
- Do you suffer from breast tenderness?
- Do you especially crave foods premenstrually?
- Do you suffer from memory loss or poor concentration?
- Do you often suffer from cyclical mood swings?
- Do you suffer from depression or low moods?
- Do you experience cyclical bloating?

If you answer 'yes' to more than 2 questions then you are showing signs of PMS. The classic time to experience these symptoms is up to 5 days before the start of your period. A few women also experience symptoms at ovulation, the midpoint of the cycle.

Symptom-free Menopause

The menopause is a process that usually takes about 10 years to complete – in most women it starts around the age of 45 and is complete by 55. Commonly called the 'change of life', it refers to the phase which leads up to the last menstrual period and more or less marks the end of reproductive life for a woman. It affects the balance of the sex hormones: the ovaries stop producing eggs, produce much less oestrogens and no progesterone.

At the menopause, less oestrogens are made because they are no longer needed to prepare the womb lining for pregnancy. As oestrogen levels fall, the menstrual flow becomes lighter and often irregular, until eventually it stops altogether. As the menopause progresses, many cycles occur in which an egg is not released. These are known as anovulatory cycles.

Symptoms of menopause include hot flushes, irregular periods, vaginal dryness, joint pains, insomnia, headaches and depression. The usual remedy prescribed by doctors is HRT. Rarely are women educated about how they can help themselves to cope with the menopause naturally.

Hot flushes may be reduced by supplementing vitamin E, vitamin C and bioflavonoids. Vitamin E also appears to help stabilise hormone levels. Using vitamin E cream locally has helped many women with vaginal dryness, as have natural oestrogen creams in the form of oestriol. Supplementing vitamins A and C, plus zinc, is also important for keeping vaginal membranes healthy. Avoiding coffee, alcohol and red wine can help improve flushes, headaches and other symptoms of menopause.

There are combination supplements available for menopausal symptoms. Make sure they contain at least the following: vitamin A 2,250mcg, vitamin D 10mcg, vitamin E 100mg, vitamin B1 25mg, B2 25mg, B3 (niacin) 50mg, B5 (pantothenic acid) 50mg, B6 50mg, B12 5mcg, folic acid 50mcg, biotin 50mcg, as well as herbs such as dong quai or schizandra. See page 99 for suggestions.

MENOPAUSE CHECK

- Are your periods becoming lighter or irregular? ☐
- Do you suffer from hot flushes? ☐
- Do you suffer from vaginal dryness? ☐
- Are you changing shape – have you gained weight either on your
  thighs and hips, or on your chest and stomach? ☐
- Do you suffer from insomnia? ☐
- Do you suffer from cyclical bloating? ☐
- Do you suffer from depression, anxiety, panic attacks or nervousness? ☐
- Do you have a reduced libido or loss of interest in sex? ☐

If you answer 'yes' to 4 or more questions then you are showing signs that you may be going through the menopause. This can be checked by a blood test arranged by your doctor.

Are You Going Through the Male Menopause?

The male menopause, known as the andropause, is finally being recognised as a real phenomenon. Many men are transforming their lives by finding remedies for their symptoms. The male mid-life crisis has been joked about now for years, as the female menopause used to be, and it is now finally getting more attention. Between the ages of 40 and 55 (it varies considerably) men can often experience quite serious symptoms, put down to 'ageing, stress or emotional problems'. These symptoms can be quite devastating as some of them hit, quite literally, 'below the belt' and at the very centre of virility and vitality.

Early symptoms can be a disappearance of the morning erection, a drop in the libido and a change in potency, i.e. erections become short-lived, hard to achieve and can disappear altogether. Also changes in the skin and the hair can occur. Skin can become drier and more wrinkly and the hair dry, dull and subject to dandruff.

Other symptoms can be a drop in energy and motivation – a desire to sit about and sleep on the couch in the evening. Depression can become a problem. Stress becomes more difficult to cope with. Other symptoms are nervousness, anxiety, night sweats and excessive sweating.

The cause of these symptoms is often quite simply a drop in the levels of the male hormone testosterone, though there can be a number of other factors involved such as poor circulation, fluctuating blood sugar levels (see Week 1, page 46), poor nutrition, diet, stress, smoking and alcohol.

Reduced libido affects both men and women and can be affected by a variety of factors including psychological and hormonal factors, disease, surgery, stress, drugs and high exposure to heavy metals. The physiological and hormonal changes that accompany stress and depression may contribute to low sexual interest by affecting the central nervous system and creating a reduction in testosterone, which is required for sexual desire. Several studies show a significant and consistent depression of blood testosterone levels in men under stress. Studies are also being undertaken to evaluate the effects of smoking on testosterone levels.

Low testosterone levels are today becoming more common due to the increasing levels of synthetic hormones (especially oestrogen-like chemicals which compete with testosterone) found in water and in the food chain (see page 103).

There are combination supplements available containing nutrients which support the male hormone system. Look out for ones which contain zinc, vitamin E, ginseng, saw palmetto and damiana.

Week 3

ANDROPAUSE CHECK

- Do you suffer from reduced libido or loss of interest in sex? ☐
- Do you suffer from impotence or reduced potency? ☐
- Do you rarely get an early morning erection? ☐
- Do you have dry skin, especially on your hands and face? ☐
- Is your hair dry, dull or lifeless? ☐
- Do you suffer from depression or low moods? ☐
- Do you suffer from fatigue or a lack of motivation? ☐
- Do you suffer from mood swings or irritability? ☐
- Do you experience memory loss or poor concentration? ☐

If you answer 'yes' to more than 3 questions, then you are showing signs that you may be going through the male andropause or suffering from a hormone imbalance.

If you think the andropause is a problem for you, do visit a doctor and have a hormone test. The saliva test, rather than the blood test, is more accurate.

The Fats of Life

Fat is good for you. Eating the right kind of fat is essential for optimal health. In fact, unless you go out of your way to eat the right kind of fat-rich foods, such as seeds, nuts and fish, the chances are that you're not getting enough good fat. Essential fats can reduce the symptoms of PMS and the menopause as well as allergies, arthritis, eczema, depression and infections, and they are actually needed to make the receptor sites – the 'ears' of body cells – to receive hormonal messages. A good intake of essential fats is vital for maintaining hormonal balance.

There are 3 main kinds of fat: saturated, monounsaturated and polyunsaturated. It is essential to have polyunsaturated fats or oils in the diet. Most authorities now agree that, of our total fat intake, no more than one-third should be saturated (hard) fat, and at least one-third should be polyunsaturated oils providing the 2 essential fats, Omega 6 and Omega 3.

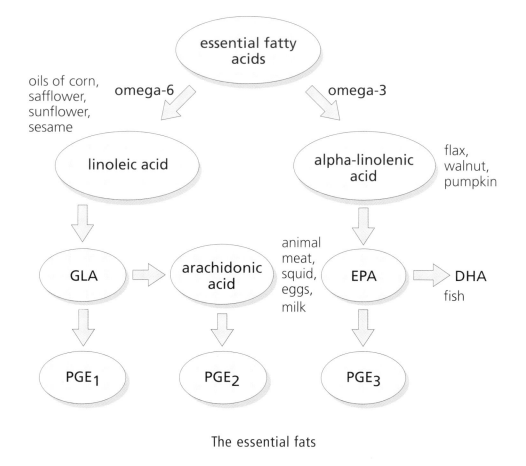

The essential fats

Essential fats cannot be made in the body, so we need to ensure that they are supplied from the diet. Most people are deficient in both Omega 6 and Omega 3 fats, though the modern diet is likely to be more deficient in Omega 3s, as we tend to eat less of them and they are more easily destroyed by cooking and processing. It is also important to avoid eating the wrong kinds of fats, which can worsen symptoms of PMS and hormone imbalance. Processed foods often contain hardened or 'hydrogenated' polyunsaturated fats or 'trans' fats, which are worse for you than saturated fat and are best avoided. Eating too much saturated fat also promotes the production of less desirable prostaglandins called PgE2, which are involved in inflammatory and clotting mechanisms in the body.

The best food sources for Omega 3 fats are fish (especially the more oily fish such as mackerel, herring or salmon) and flax seeds (also known as linseeds) and their oil. Symptoms of deficiency include dry skin, inflammatory health problems, water retention, tingling in the arms or legs, high blood pressure, infections, poor memory, lack of co-ordination, and PMS and menopausal problems. You can also buy Omega 3 fats in supplementation form as fish oil capsules – look for capsules which contain 400mg or more of EPA and DHA.

Omega 6 fats come exclusively from seeds and their oils. The best seeds, and their oils, are pumpkin, sunflower, safflower and sesame. These oils relax blood vessels and keep the blood thin, which improves heavy periods; they lower blood pressure, reduce water retention, decrease inflammation and pain including period pains, improve immunity and help insulin to work, which is good for maintaining blood sugar balance and therefore sugar cravings.

Gamma-linolenic acid, or GLA, is one of the most powerful Omega 6 fats. It is converted inside the body from linoleic acid in seeds (see page 95), and has a special role in hormone balance. GLA often becomes deficient because the body loses the ability to make this conversion from Omega 6 to GLA. This is caused by eating too many of the wrong fats, i.e. hydrogenated, trans- or saturated fats, or by deficiencies of certain minerals or vitamins, e.g. magnesium, zinc or B6, needed to make the conversion.

Deficiency signs include PMS, eczema, dry skin, excessive thirst, breast tenderness and lumpiness, irritability, dry eyes and hot flushes. Evening primrose oil and borage oil are the richest known sources of GLA. The ideal intake is probably around 150mg of GLA a day, or double this if you have PMS or other hormonal problems.

ESSENTIAL FATS CHECK

- Do you have dry skin and/or eczema?
- Do you have a poor memory?
- Do you have dandruff?
- Are you often thirsty?
- Do you suffer from PMS or breast tenderness?
- Do you suffer from dry eyes?
- Do you have inflammatory health problems, e.g. arthritis?
- Do you have high blood pressure or high blood lipids?

If you have answered 'yes' to more than 3 questions then you are very likely to be deficient in essential fats.

The Velvet Hand Test

- Gently stroke the skin on the outside of your hand using the index finger of the opposite hand. How does it feel?

- If it is rough or scaly you are probably deficient in essential fats.

- During this week, you will be taking a tablespoon of a cold-pressed, organic oil seed blend and a heaped tablespoon of ground seeds a day. Notice the difference in your Velvet Hand Test by the end of the week.

To achieve an optimal intake of essential fats, you need to eat around a heaped tablespoon of seeds a day. Since you require both Omega 3 and Omega 6 oils, your daily seed intake should include some flax, pumpkin or hemp seeds.

In practical terms, an ideal mix would be half flax seeds, with the remaining half made up of sesame, sunflower, hemp and pumpkin seeds. Since some of these seeds are quite tough, you will get more nutrients by grinding them in a coffee grinder and then sprinkling them on your morning cereal, or into soups, salads or casseroles.

Essential fats are easily oxidised and therefore lose their nutritional value if heated or stored too long, especially if exposed to light. So the best way to protect the oils in seeds is to keep them in a tightly sealed glass jar in the fridge.

The Hormone Helpers

Hormone-like substances abound in natural foods. This is hardly surprising, since hormones are, after all, made from food components. However, the extent to which foods, rich in certain phytonutrients, influence hormone balance and health has only recently been recognised.

Phyto-oestrogens – Friend or Foe?

Oestrogen-like plant compounds are often called phyto-oestrogens (phyto = plant). At first glance, given the health problems associated with oestrogen dominance, one might think that eating foods rich in phyto-oestrogens might be bad news. If anything, the reverse seems to be true. Soya products, rich in phyto-oestrogens, are reputed to protect against breast and prostate cancer, which are notably low among communities with a soya-based diet. This is because phyto-oestrogens may lock on to and block the body's oestrogen receptors, thereby making it harder for harmful chemicals to disrupt hormone signals. In this way, these phytonutrients may act more like hormone regulators. Since mankind has been exposed to these plant chemicals for millennia, it is safe to assume that we have adapted to deal with these compounds in the kind of quantities to which we are exposed by eating natural foods.

Nature's Hormone Helpers

Soya products and tofu are both excellent sources of isoflavones, which are powerful phyto-oestrogens. Isoflavones are known to decrease the risk of hormone-related cancers, including breast and prostatic cancer, and also reduce menopausal symptoms, especially hot flushes. Two particular isoflavones have been identified – genistein and diadzein. Tofu, a curd made from the soya bean, is the richest source of isoflavones.

Citrus fruits, wheat, alfalfa, hops, oats, fennel, celery and rhubarb all contain phyto-oestrogens. There is a small amount of evidence that these foods may help to balance hormones and could play a part in helping to reduce symptoms associated with hormonal imbalance.

Phytonutrient Herbs

Many herbs which help balance hormones are now available as supplements. These include:

Agnus castus The plant *Vitex aqnus castus* has a long history of use for women's problems. Traditionally it has been used to relieve premenstrual and menopausal problems.

Black cohosh, dong quai and wild yam These all have progesterone-favourable effects on the body. Yams are especially rich in diosgenin, from which progesterone can be made in the laboratory. We cannot, however, turn these phytonutrients into progesterone itself, so while these plants may help to balance hormones, they do not replace the need for progesterone in a person who is progesterone-deficient.

Ginseng and licorice These are considered to contain quite powerful 'adapto-gens', substances that help restore hormonal balance. For example, licorice appears to potentiate oestrogen when levels are too low and inhibit oestrogen when levels are too high. Ginseng is a classic herbal remedy for increasing one's ability to deal with stress. Both have widespread uses for a number of hormonal conditions, probably because adrenal hormones and sex hormones are very closely related, with the adrenal glands producing small amounts of sex hormones.

Damiana and saw palmetto These are probably the 2 most popular herbs for male hormonal health. Saw palmetto gained notoriety in the treatment of prostatitis, enlargement of the prostate gland, a condition frequently suffered by men over 40. Damiana, which has a testosterone-like effect, has long been asso-ciated with increasing male potency. These herbs, together with ginseng, are often included in male herbal tonics.

In summary, the inclusion of the right phytonutrient foods and herbs may help the body to adapt, thus restoring and maintaining hormonal balance. Many supplements designed to support female or male health contain combinations of these herbs and are likely to be beneficial (see page 213).

Week 3

HORMONE-BALANCING **Action Plan**

DOs

■ Eat 1 heaped tablespoon of ground seeds daily to increase your levels of essential fats, or take 1 tablespoon of a cold-pressed, organic oil blend (see page 97) on salads, in soups or cereal, or neat with some juice. Do not cook with this oil.

■ Eat 2 servings of beans, chickpeas or lentils daily – make sure at least one of these servings is from soya.

■ Eat whole organic food as much as you can to avoid hormone disruptors (see page 103).

And as always . . .

1 heaped tablespoon of ground seeds or 1 tablespoon of cold-pressed seed oil.

2 servings of beans, lentils, quinoa, tofu (soya), or 'seed' vegetables.

3 pieces of fresh fruit such as apples, pears, bananas, berries, melon or citrus fruit.

4 servings of wholegrains such as rice, millet, rye, oats, corn or quinoa.

5 servings of dark green, leafy and root vegetables such as watercress, carrots, sweet potatoes, broccoli, spinach, green beans, peas and peppers.

6 glasses of water, diluted juices, herb or fruit teas.

7 Eat whole, organic, raw food as much as you can.

8 Avoid any form of sugar, white, refined or processed food with chemical additives.

9 Avoid all stimulants – coffee, tea, cigarettes.

10 Relax during your meal and chew your food well.

DON'Ts

■ Avoid all 'hydrogenated' fats and 'trans' fats, eating only 'non' or 'unhydrogenated' margarines.

■ Avoid all meat except for free-range chicken.

■ Avoid all dairy products.

■ Limit your alcohol intake to no more than 2 units on 2 nights during this week, ideally red wine.

HORMONE-BALANCING Menus

Below are some meal recommendations for Week 3. You can of course use or adapt recipes from other weeks which comply with the current 'Dos and Don'ts'.

Breakfast
Choose from:
● Ultimate Power Breakfast (page 174)
● Get Up & Go (page 213) blended with skimmed or soya milk and a banana
● Simple Fruit Muesli (page 177)
● Oat Porridge (page 176)

Other recipes can be taken from *The Optimum Nutrition Cookbook* (Piatkus, 1999), which I co-authored with Judy Ridgway.

Lunch
Choose from:
● Smoked Tofu on Oriental Glass Noodles with Shredded Vegetables (page 191)
● Rocket Salad with Chickpeas in Tahini Dressing (page 188)
● Chunky Bean and Kale Soup (page 188)

Other recommended recipes, taken from *The Optimum Nutrition Cookbook*, include: Spaghetti Pomodoro with Olives; Warm Mackerel Salad with Avocado and Mango served with Honey-toasted Sunflower Seeds; Beetroot and Tahini Special Sandwich; Jacket Potato with Tofu Topping.

Week 3

Dinner

Choose from:

- Roasted Chicory and Courgettes with Salsa Picante and Bulgar (page 194)
- Grilled Carrot and Tofu Cakes with Red Peppers and Fennel (page 195)
- Spicy Mackerel with Couscous (page 198)

Other recommended recipes, taken from *The Optimum Nutrition Cookbook*, include: Thai Noodle Salad, Oriental Seafood with Sushi Rice, Vegetarian Chilli with Taco Shells and Green Salad, Vegetarian Kebabs with Barbecue Sauce and Brown Rice.

HORMONE-BALANCING Supplements

As always	BREAKFAST	LUNCH	DINNER
Multi-vitamin/mineral	2		
Vitamin C 1,000mg	1		

Add			
Essential Balance (see page 213)	1 tablespoon		

Optional

- Take a PMS prevention combination supplement (see page 90), if you have symptoms of PMS.
- Take a combination supplement for the menopause (see page 92), if you have menopausal symptoms.
- Take a combination supplement for symptoms of the andropause (see page 93) if you are a man having symptoms of hormonal imbalance.

Optional to continue	BREAKFAST	LUNCH	DINNER
Chromium 200mcg	1		
Digestive enzymes	1	1	1
Herbal Aloe Detox	1 tablespoon		1 tablespoon

HORMONE-BALANCING **Awareness Exercise**

Avoiding the Chemicals

We are all exposed, unwittingly, to hormone-disrupting chemicals. Use this week as a chance to reduce your exposure by switching to alternative foods, toiletries, household products and packaging.

The key chemicals to avoid are:

- **Pesticides** – DDT, DDE, endosulfan, methoxychlor, heptachlor, toxaphene, dieldrin, lindane, atrazine.

- **Plastic compounds** – alkyphenols, such as nonylphenol and octylphenol; biphenolic compounds, such as bisphenol A; phthalates.

- **Industrial compounds** – some PCBs (polychlorinated biphenyls), dioxin, plus those listed for plastics.

- **Pharmaceutical drugs** – synthetic oestrogens, such as DES.

- **Cosmetics** – parabens.

- **Foods** – butylated hydroxyanisole (BHA, an antioxidant).

- **Check your bathroom products** for these chemicals. If you find them included switch to a different brand.

- **Check your washing-up liquid, dishwasher and washer detergents.** If you find any of these chemicals switch to another brand, such as Ecover, available in all health food stores.

The more you eat organic, the lower your risk of exposure to hormone-disrupting chemicals. Particularly important to avoid are non-organic grains, breads and cereals, since these often contain higher levels of pesticides and herbicides.

- **Find a source of organic flour, bread and cereals** by checking in your supermarket or healthfood shop.
- **Find a source of organic fruit and vegetables** – ask your local healthfood shop for a recommendation if they do not actually sell fresh produce themselves.

Fatty and liquid foods that are exposed to soft, flexible plastics can absorb hormone-disrupting 'plasticisers'. Until the plastics industry stop using known

Week 3

hormone-disrupting 'plasticisers' your best bet is to limit exposure as follows:

- **Choose fruit juices and other drinks in glass or hard plastic** rather than cartons lined with soft plastic.

- **Choose alternatives to canned products with an inner lining of plastic.** Check the inside of any canned foods you buy frequently.

- **Minimise plastic packaging** by buying fewer foods in plastic, recycling plastic bags, storing food in paper bags and wrapping food in greaseproof paper.

WEEK 3 Psychocalisthenics Exercises

Now you are familiar with the routines for Weeks 1 and 2, it is time to add another 3 exercises.

Shoulder Rolls

Foot position 2 foot-widths

Breathing *Inhale*, roll shoulders in 3 backward circles, 3 counts: *Exhale*, drop shoulders, 1 count

Repeat ×6

Points to note The inhalation is continuous throughout the Shoulder Rolls. At the end of the inhalation, the shoulders are up toward the ears, not back. The shoulders drop down with the exhale. Keep the neck and torso still, relaxing your face and isolating the movement in your shoulders.

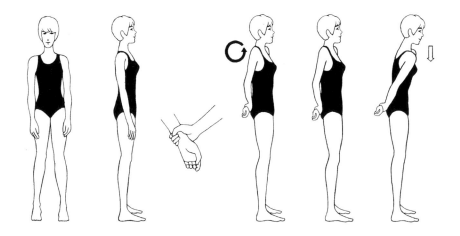

Arm Circles

Foot position 3 foot-widths

Breathing *Inhale*, make 3 circles in, up and around, 3 counts: *Exhale*, make 3 circles down, out and around, 3 counts

Repeat ×6

Points to note The arms are like moving tree branches, and the body is stable like the tree trunk. The 3 foot-width stance is the position of strength. The knees are unlocked. With the circles, don't let the arms go behind the vertical plane of the body, and avoid allowing the circles to extend below the horizontal plane of the shoulders. Feel the muscle movements in the upper back, shoulders, upper arms, and sides of the neck.

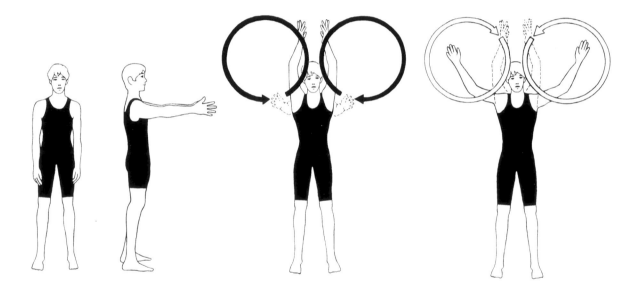

Week 3

Hand Circles

Foot position 2 foot-widths

Breathing *Hands in 'bird's beak' position: Inhale*, make 3 circles out, down, and around, 3 counts: *Exhale*, make 3 circles in, down and around, 3 counts

Repeat ×6

Points to note The fingertips and thumbtips touch throughout the rotation. Make as smooth and circular a movement as possible. Watch each of your hands from time to time, monitoring their movement. Relax your shoulders and keep your elbows relaxed at your sides.

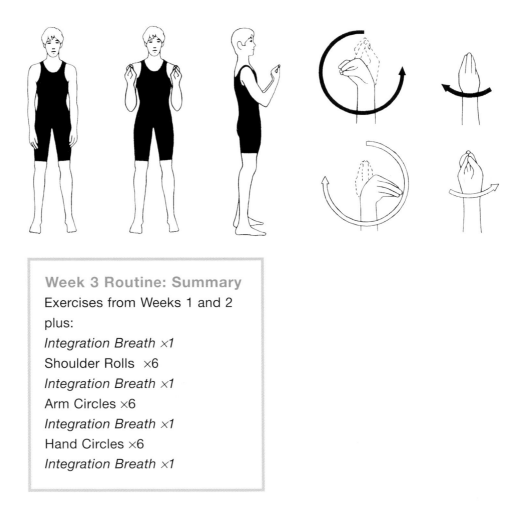

Week 3 Routine: Summary
Exercises from Weeks 1 and 2 plus:
Integration Breath ×1
Shoulder Rolls ×6
Integration Breath ×1
Arm Circles ×6
Integration Breath ×1
Hand Circles ×6
Integration Breath ×1

You are now halfway to superhealth. You will find the programme beginning to get easier as your health levels improve.

WEEK 4

DETOX FOR SUPERHEALTH

Why Detoxify?

Throughout the centuries, health experts have extolled the value of spring-cleaning the body. Just as you need a holiday, a break from your work, your body needs a break from its work. One of the traditional methods for purifying the body is fasting. The fact that many people report feeling so much more vital after fasting is a testimony to the fact that making energy is as much a result of improving the body's ability to detoxify as it is about eating the right foods.

However, not everyone feels better from fasting and not always right away. A common occurrence is the so-called 'healing crisis', when a person feels worse for a few days and then feels better. What we are learning about detoxification processes suggests that some people may be experiencing a crisis, not a healing crisis. Once the body starts to liberate and eliminate toxic material, if the liver isn't up to the job symptoms of intoxication can result. So modern-day detox regimes tend to use modified fasts in which the person is given a low-toxin diet, plus plenty of the key nutrients needed to speed up the body's ability to detoxify. Doing this once a year, for a week, can greatly increase your energy levels.

Chronic fatigue, multiple allergies, frequent headaches, sensitivity to chemicals and environmental pollutants, chronic digestive problems, muscle aches, autism, schizophrenia, drug reactions and Gulf War Syndrome are just some of the conditions that can be caused by a breakdown in the body's ability to detoxify.

Once too many toxins and large molecules start 'gate-crashing' through the digestive tract, the body has to work overtime to detoxify and deal with them. Before long, the body's ability to detoxify all the uninvited guests starts to weaken, resulting in compromised liver function. By this stage even the slightest increase in toxins results in a whole host of symptoms such as fatigue, drowsiness, headaches, body aches and inflammation. For example, when we exercise, muscles tend to produce a toxin called lactic acid which is what can make them a bit stiff the next day. This is no problem normally, but if a person's detox potential is poor even a brisk walk can trigger symptoms.

Prevention, however, is better than cure, so if you are basically healthy and want to promote and maintain optimal liver function the best advice is to cut down on your intake of toxic substances, eat an optimal diet and take a balanced nutrition supplement programme.

CHECK YOUR DETOX POTENTIAL

Complete this questionnaire to discover whether you need to improve your detoxification potential.

- Do you often suffer from headaches or migraine?

- Do you sometimes have watery or itchy eyes or swollen, red or sticky eyelids?

- Do you have dark circles under your eyes?

- Do you sometimes have itchy ears, earache, ear infections, drainage from ears or ringing in ears?

- Do you often suffer from excessive mucus, a stuffy nose or sinus problems?

- Do you suffer from acne or skin rashes or hives?

- Do you sweat a lot and have a strong body odour?

- Do you sometimes have joint or muscle aches or pains?

- Do you have a sluggish metabolism and find it hard to lose weight, or are you underweight and find it hard to gain weight?

- Do you often suffer from frequent or urgent urination?

- Do you suffer from nausea or vomiting?
- Do you often have a bitter taste in your mouth or a furry tongue?
- Do you have a strong reaction to alcohol?
- Do you suffer from bloating?
- Does coffee stay in your system for a long time?

- If you answer 'yes' to 7 or more questions you need to improve your detox potential.
- If you answer 'yes' to between 4 and 7 questions you are beginning to show signs of poor detoxification and need to improve your detox potential.
- If you answer 'yes' to less than 4 questions, you are unlikely to have a problem with detoxification.

How the Body Detoxifies

If eating the right food is one side of the coin, detoxification is the other. It's all too easy to think that food is good for you. Of course it is, but the truth is that almost all food contains toxins as well as nutrients. So too do air and water.

From a chemical perspective, much of what goes on in the body is that substances are broken down, built up and turned from one thing into another. A good 80 per cent of this involves detoxifying potentially harmful substances. Much of this is done by the liver, which represents a clearing house, able to recognise millions of potentially harmful chemicals and transform them into something harmless or prepare them for elimination. It is the chemical brain of the body – recycling, regenerating and detoxifying in order to maintain your health.

These external or exo-toxins represent just a small part of what the liver has to deal with; many toxins are made within the body from otherwise harmless molecules. Every breath and every action can generate toxins. These internally created or endo-toxins have to be disarmed in just the same way as exo-toxins do. Whether a substance is bad for you depends as much on your ability to detoxify it as its inherent toxic properties.

How the liver detoxifies can be split into two stages. The first, known as Phase 1, is akin to getting your garbage ready for collection, while Phase 2 collects and

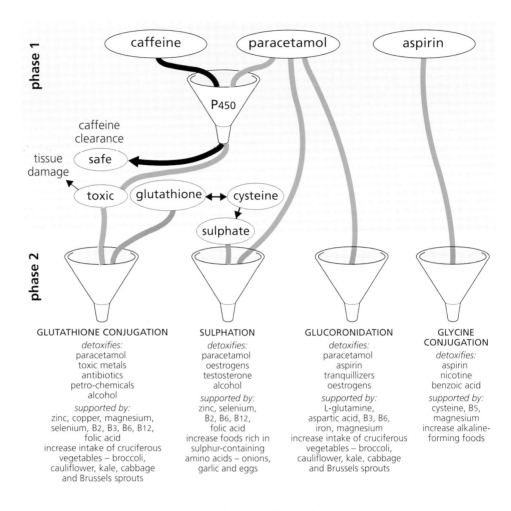

caffeine   paracetamol   aspirin

P450

caffeine clearance

tissue damage

safe

toxic   glutathione ↔ cysteine

sulphate

GLUTATHIONE CONJUGATION
detoxifies:
paracetamol
toxic metals
antibiotics
petro-chemicals
alcohol
supported by:
zinc, copper, magnesium,
selenium, B2, B3, B6, B12,
folic acid
increase intake of cruciferous
vegetables – broccoli,
cauliflower, kale, cabbage
and Brussels sprouts

SULPHATION
detoxifies:
paracetamol
oestrogens
testosterone
alcohol
supported by:
zinc, selenium,
B2, B6, B12,
folic acid
increase foods rich in
sulphur-containing
amino acids – onions,
garlic and eggs

GLUCORONIDATION
detoxifies:
paracetamol
aspirin
tranquillizers
oestrogens
supported by:
L-glutamine,
aspartic acid, B3, B6,
iron, magnesium
increase intake of cruciferous
vegetables – broccoli,
cauliflower, kale, cabbage
and Brussels sprouts

**GLYCINE
CONJUGATION**
detoxifies:
aspirin
nicotine
benzoic acid
supported by:
cysteine, B5,
magnesium
increase alkaline-
forming foods

How the liver detoxifies

gets rid of the garbage. Phase 1 doesn't actually eliminate anything, just prepares it for elimination, making it easier to pick up.

The end-products of Phase 1 are often transformed by 'sticking' things on to them in a process called conjugation, and then eliminated. Some toxins have glutathione stuck to them (this is called glutathione conjugation). This is how we detoxify paracetamol, for example. In cases of overdose, a person is given glutathione to mop up the highly destructive toxins generated by Phase 1 detoxification of this drug.

Other toxins have sulphur stuck to them in a process called sulphation. This is the fate of many steroid hormones, neurotransmitters and, once again, paracetamol. The sulphur comes directly from food. Garlic, onions and eggs, for example, are good sources of sulphur-containing amino acids, so a lack of these can create a problem. Others have carbon compounds, called methyl groups, stuck to them (this is called methylation). Lead and arsenic are detoxified in this way.

Too Many Toxins or Not Enough Nutrients?

Substances which interfere with proper liver function include caffeine, alcohol, recreational and medicinal drugs, the pill and HRT, dioxins, cigarette smoke, exhaust fumes, high-protein diets, organophosphate fertilisers, paint fumes, saturated fat, steroid hormones and charcoal-barbecued meat.

The proper functioning of Phase 1 and Phase 2 also depends on a long list of nutrients, including vitamins B2, B3, B6, B12, folic acid, glutathione and flavonoids, plus a generous supply of antioxidant nutrients to deal with the oxidants (see pages 112–15 on antioxidants and oxidants). When these biochemical pathways don't work properly, due to overload or a lack of nutrients, the body generates harmful toxins.

Liver Problems or Health Problems?

Having a liver's-eye view on disease processes often sheds new light on the health problems and solutions of the late twentieth century. Just about any allergic, inflammatory or metabolic disorder may involve or create sub-optimum liver function, including eczema, asthma, chronic fatigue, chronic infections, inflammatory bowel disorders, multiple sclerosis, rheumatoid arthritis and hormone imbalances.

The brain is not able to disarm a wide range of toxins – it depends on the liver to do a chemical clean-up of the blood before it gets there. So toxic overload of the liver has dire consequences for brain and nervous system function. Autism, schizophrenia and memory loss are all associated with poor liver function. A classic example is alcoholism. Once the liver can't deal with the quantity of alcohol consumed, the brain is left unprotected, which is why brain damage, dementia and mental illness are some particularly unpleasant consequences of chronic alcohol abuse. Liver problems usually lead to accumulation of fat in the liver, which can be responsible for 'fatty liver' or 'sluggish liver' associated with excess alcohol consumption. Alcohol is definitely no friend to your liver.

The good news is that, with a good diet, lifestyle, regular detoxification and the right supplements you can restore and maintain optimal liver function.

Week 4

Week 4

Protect Yourself with Antioxidants

We are threatened by internal toxins as well as external ones. For example, oxygen is the basis of all plant and animal life. It is our most important nutrient, needed by every cell every second of every day. Without it we cannot release the energy in food which drives all body processes. Oxygen is also chemically reactive and highly dangerous. In normal biochemical reactions oxygen can become unstable and capable of 'oxidising' neighbouring molecules. This can lead to cellular damage which triggers cancer, inflammation, arterial damage and ageing.

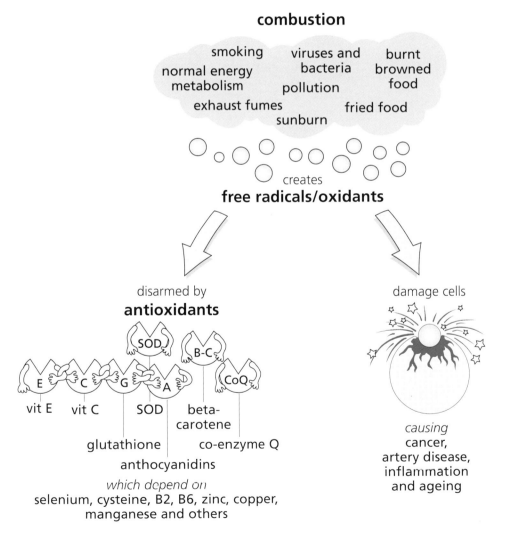

Oxidants and antioxidants

Known as 'oxidants', this equivalent of 'nuclear waste' must be disarmed to remove the danger, as they are the most dangerous toxin of all. Oxidants are made in all combustion processes, including smoking, exhaust fumes, radiation, fried or barbecued food and normal body processes. Chemicals capable of disarming oxidants are termed 'antioxidants'. Some are known essential nutrients, like vitamins A, C, E and beta-carotene. Others are not essential as such, like bioflavonoids, anthocyanidins, pycnogenol and over 100 other recently identified protectors found in common foods.

The balance between your intake of anti-oxidants and exposure to oxidants may literally be the difference between life and death. You can tip the scales in your favour by simple changes to your diet and taking antioxidant supplements.

Antioxidants – the Main Players

Vitamins A, C and E

Vitamin A comes in two forms: retinol from animals, and beta-carotene from plants. Of these two, beta-carotene is the more powerful antioxidant. Vitamin C, which is water-soluble, and vitamin E, fat-soluble, are synergistic: together they can protect both the tissues and fluids in the body. What's more, when vitamin E has 'disarmed' an oxidant, it can be reloaded by vitamin C, so their combined presence in the diet and the body has a synergistic effect. Combining all three is better still and has been proven to more than halve cancer risk. They have also been shown to protect against Alzheimer's, cataracts and heart disease.

Beta-carotene is found in red/orange/yellow vegetables and fruits. Vitamin C is also rich in vegetables and fruits eaten raw, as heat rapidly destroys it. Vitamin E is found in 'seed' foods, including nuts, seeds and their oils, but also vegetables like peas, broad beans, corn, wholegrains – all of which are classified as seed foods. Eating sweet potatoes, carrots, watercress, peas and broccoli frequently is a great way to increase your antioxidant levels, provided, of course, you don't fry them. Another great food is watermelon. The flesh is high in beta-carotene and vitamin C. The seeds are high in vitamin E, and in antioxidant minerals zinc and selenium.

Zinc and Selenium

These are two key antioxidant minerals – they are needed to activate two main antioxidant enzymes: glutathione peroxidase, which is selenium-dependent, and superoxide dismutase, which is dependent on zinc. Seeds and seafood are the best all-round dietary sources of selenium and zinc.

Anthocyanidins

These are powerful antioxidants from the flavonoid family, which account for the different colours of many plants, for example, purple, red, orange, yellow and green. Plants all contain different types of anthocyanidins – so make sure your diet is naturally colourful. A diet rich in fruits and vegetables can deliver up to a gram of these important nutrients a day and may be as significant in their health-promoting properties as vitamins and minerals. Anthocyanidins (sometimes called anthocyans) provide dramatic colours in foods, such as those in black grapes, blueberries and cranberries. Grape seeds, bilberries, cranberries and pine bark (pycnogenol) are especially rich sources. They are even more powerful when combined with other key antioxidants, especially glutathione-related compounds, which they help to recycle (see page 112).

Glutathione

Glutathione is the key ingredient in the antioxidant enzyme glutathione peroxidase, also dependent on selenium. This enzyme helps to detoxify the body, protecting against car exhaust, carcinogens, infections, excessive alcohol and toxic metals. White meat, tuna, lentils, beans, nuts and seeds are particularly rich in glutathione and have been shown to boost the immune system as well as increasing antioxidant power. Glutathione is perhaps the most important antioxidant, protecting against the harmful effects of carcinogens, especially oxidants and radiation. The body can also make glutathione from the amino acid cysteine.

CoQ10

CoQ is a vital antioxidant helping to protect cells from carcinogens and also helping to recycle vitamin E. CoQ's magical properties lie in its ability to improve the cell's use of oxygen. CoQ10 works by controlling the flow of oxygen, making the production of energy most efficient, and preventing damage caused by these oxidants. CoQ is found in meat, fish, nuts and seeds.

Lipoic Acid

This is a sulphur-containing vitamin-like substance which has very effective antioxidant properties. As an antioxidant it is particularly useful because it is one of the few that is both water- and fat-soluble, which means it can protect a wider range of molecules than, say, just vitamin C or vitamin E. Foods said to be high in lipoic acid are liver and yeast.

Antioxidant Supplements

It is wise to make sure your daily supplement programme contains significant quantities of antioxidants, especially if you are older, live in a polluted city or have any other unavoidable exposure to oxidants.

The easiest way to do this is to take a comprehensive antioxidant supplement, in addition to a good multi-vitamin and mineral. Most reputable supplement companies produce formulas containing a combination of the following nutrients: vitamin A, beta-carotene, vitamin E, vitamin C, zinc, selenium, glutathione, plus plant-based antioxidants such as anthocyanidins from a source such as bilberry or pycnogenol. The kind of total supplementary intake (which may come in part from a multi-vitamin and extra vitamin C) to aim for is shown below:

Vitamin A (retinol/beta-carotene)	2,500mgRE (7500iu) to 6,600mgRE (20000iu)
Glutathione (reduced)	25mg to 75mg
Vitamin E	66mg (100iu) to 330mg (500iu)
Vitamin C	1,000mg to 3,000mg
CoQ10	10mg to 50mg
Lipoic acid	10mg to 50mg
Anthocyanidin source	50mg to 250mg
Selenium	30mcg to 100mcg
Zinc	10mg to 20mg

Week 4

DETOX **Action Plan**

DOs

- Begin your detox at the weekend or during a time when you don't have too much going on.

- Walk for at least 15 minutes every day.

- Drink at least 2 litres of purified, distilled, filtered or bottled water a day. You can also drink dandelion coffee or herb teas.

- Have ½ a pint of fruit or vegetable juice – either carrot and apple juice (you can buy these separately and combine them with one-third water) with grated ginger, or fresh watermelon juice a day. The flesh of the watermelon is high in beta-carotene and vitamin C. The seeds are high in vitamin E, and in antioxidant minerals zinc and selenium. You can make a great antioxidant cocktail by blending flesh and seeds in a blender.

● Eat in abundance:

Fruit – the most beneficial fruits with the highest detox potential include fresh apricots, all types of berries, cantaloupe, citrus fruits, kiwi, papaya, peaches, mango, melons, red grapes.

Vegetables – especially good for detoxification are artichokes, peppers, beet-root, Brussels sprouts, broccoli, red cabbage, carrots, cauliflower, cucumber, kale, pumpkin, spinach, sweet potato, tomato, watercress and bean and seed sprouts.

● Eat in moderation:

Grains – brown rice, corn, millet, quinoa – small portions which make up to more than a quarter of each meal.

Fish – salmon, mackerel, sardines, tuna – not more than once a day.

Oils – use extra-virgin olive oil for cooking and in place of butter, and cold-pressed seed oils for dressing.

Nuts and seeds – 1 handful a day of raw, unsalted nuts and seeds should be included. Choose from almonds, Brazils, hazelnuts, pecans, pumpkin seeds, sunflower seeds, sesame seeds and flax seeds.

And as always . . .

1 heaped tablespoon of ground seeds or 1 tablespoon of cold-pressed seed oil.

2 servings of beans, lentils, quinoa, tofu (soya), or 'seed' vegetables.

3 pieces of fresh fruit such as apples, pears, bananas, berries, melon or citrus fruit.

4 servings of wholegrains such as rice, millet, rye, oats, corn or quinoa.

5 servings of dark green, leafy and root vegetables such as watercress, carrots, sweet potatoes, broccoli, spinach, green beans, peas and peppers.

6 glasses of water, diluted juices, herb or fruit teas.

7 Eat whole, organic, raw food as much as you can.

8 Avoid any form of sugar, white, refined or processed food with chemical additives.

9 Avoid all stimulants – coffee, tea, cigarettes.

10 Relax during your meal and chew your food well.

DON'Ts

■ Avoid all wheat products.

■ Avoid all meat and dairy produce – milk and all dairy products, eggs and meat.

■ Avoid salt – and any foods containing it.

■ Avoid hydrogenated fats.

■ Avoid artificial sweeteners.

■ Avoid food additives and preservatives.

■ Avoid alcohol.

■ Avoid fried foods.

■ Avoid spices.

■ Avoid dried fruit.

■ Limit potatoes to 1 portion every other day.

■ Limit bananas to 1 every other day.

DETOX Menus

Below are some meal recommendations for Week 4. You can of course use or adapt recipes from other weeks which comply to the current 'Dos and Don'ts'.

Breakfast

(Replace dairy foods with soya milk and yoghurt or rice milk.)

Choose from:

• Ultimate Power Breakfast (page 174)
• Get Up & Go (page 213) blended with skimmed or soya milk and a banana
• Millet or Rice Flake Porridge (page 177)
• Berry Booster (page 175)

Other recipes can be taken from *The Optimum Nutrition Cookbook* (Piatkus, 1999), which I co-authored with Judy Ridgway.

Lunch

Choose from:

- Brussels Sprouts and Nut Salad (page 180)
- Red Cabbage and Mixed Vegetable Salad with Tofu (page 180)
- Steam-Fried Vegetables with Green Curry Paste (page 182)

Other recommended recipes, taken from *The Optimum Nutrition Cookbook*, include: Quinoa Pilaf with Chickpeas and Dried Fruits; Spanish Rice with Fennel; Celery and Apple Soup with Ginger; Jacket Potato with Tofu Topping.

Dinner

Choose from:

- Thai Baked Fish with Steam-fried Vegetables (page 203)
- Garden Paella (page 200)
- Salmon and Monkfish Kebabs with Coriander and Sunflower Seed Pesto (page 193)

Other recommended recipes, taken from *The Optimum Nutrition Cookbook*, include: Chestnut Hotpot with Beansprout Salad; Warm Avocado, Arame, Rice and Quinoa Salad with Rainbow Roots; Baked Aubergines with Peppers, Quinoa and Broccoli Salsa; Grilled Sea Bass on a Bed of Swiss Chard.

DETOX Supplements

As always	BREAKFAST	LUNCH	DINNER
Multi-vitamin/mineral	2		
Vitamin C 1,000mg	1		

Add			
Antioxidant Complex	1		1

Optional			
MSM 1,000mg	1		1

■ Take MSM if you scored 7 or more in the questionnaire on page 108.

Optional to continue	BREAKFAST	LUNCH	DINNER
Chromium 200mcg	1		
Digestive enzymes	1	1	1
Herbal Aloe Detox	1 tablespoon		1 tablespoon
Essential Balance	1 tablespoon		

DETOX Awareness Exercise

Detoxify Your Life

Detoxification is about eliminating what is unnecessary. As you do this on the inside, by detoxifying your body, you can also do it on the outside, by detoxifying your environment.

- **Spring-clean a room in your house or workplace** – perhaps your living room, bedroom, study or office. Go through each drawer and cupboard and throw away that which you never use. If in doubt, throw it out. Now open the windows and clean your room thoroughly. Buy some flowers or a plant for your room and then burn some incense or aromatherapy oil.

- **Have a massage** – the body stores toxins, tension and negative emotions. A good massage helps to restore balance. Regular massage is part of my ongoing strategy for superhealth. My favourite type of massage is called Chua Ka, which you can learn and give to yourself or your friends and partner.

- **Practice the following visualisation every evening, before bed:** Lie down in a quiet place, place a glass of distilled, filtered or bottled water beside you.

  Relax the muscles in your legs, buttocks, abdomen, back, shoulders, arms, neck and face. Let all the tensions of the day subside and bring your attention to your breathing.

  Let your inhalation naturally become a little deeper and your exhalation a little longer. Practice Dia–Kath Breathing (see page 59) for 9 breaths.

  As you take 3 slow breaths, imagine that your entire body becomes completely hollow.

  As you take 3 slow breaths imagine your entire body becomes filled with water, as pure as a mountain stream. Feel the water regenerate all your cells, removing toxins and filling them with vitality.

  Bring your attention back to your surroundings and sit up. Slowly drink the glass of water. With each sip taste the water, and be aware that the major constituent of your body is water. Be aware that this water is purifying and detoxifying your body.

WEEK 4 **Psychocalisthenics Exercises**

Here are 6 new exercises to add to the *Psychocalisthenics* routines you learnt in the first 3 weeks.

Windmill

Foot position 1½ foot-widths

Breathing *Inhale*, circle backward, 6 counts: *Hold breath*, 1 count: *Exhale*, circle forward, 3 counts: *Rest*, 1 count

Repeat ×3

Points to note Bend your knees and lean your torso forward. Check your stance in a mirror if possible, making sure your head, neck and spine are in a line making a 90 degree angle with the line of your thighs. Look at a place on the ground about 3 feet in front of your feet. Let your arms dangle and swing loosely with their own weight. Begin to rotate your knees and hips from side to side, and notice how your arms swing correspondingly. Then take the arm swings up and over to make a full rotation and start the exercise. In this way you will have originated the movement in the knees and hips. Imagine the arms as chains flung into orbit, and feel the tingling in your fingertips.

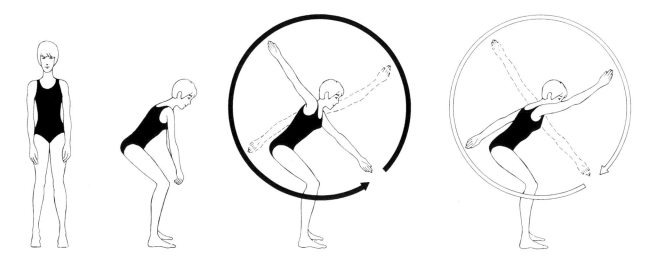

Scythe

Foot position 3 foot-widths

Breathing *Inhale*, left, 1 count: *Exhale*, centre, 1 count: *Inhale*, right, 1 count: *Exhale*, centre, 1 count

Repeat ×6

Points to note Raise your arms to shoulder level, keeping the shoulders and neck relaxed and the head up. Throw both arms as far behind you to each side as possible, keeping the arms roughly parallel. This stretches the muscles in the middle and lower parts of the back. Let the hips, torso and head follow the movement of the arms. Focus your sight on your fingertips. Each inhalation and exhalation is swiftly filling and emptying your lungs as fully as possible. Avoid shortening the breaths. The breath moves the exercise.

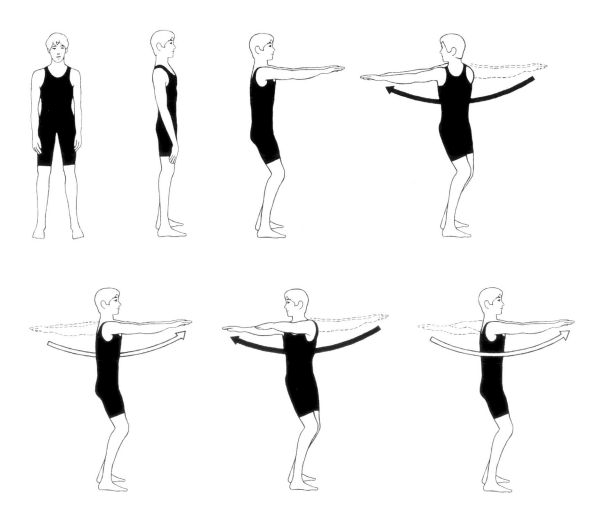

Head Circles

Foot position 2 foot-widths

Breathing *Inhale*, circle up and back, 2 counts: *Exhale*, circle down and forward, 2 counts

Repeat left ×6; right ×6

Points to note The shoulders are relaxed and the knees unlocked. Your arms hang relaxed at your sides, with your fingertips resting lightly against your thighs and not moving up and down with the movement of your head. Isolate the movement in your head and neck by not allowing your torso to move as well. Feel the movement of the muscle groups all around the neck. On the inhale, avoid straining and forcing your head too far back.

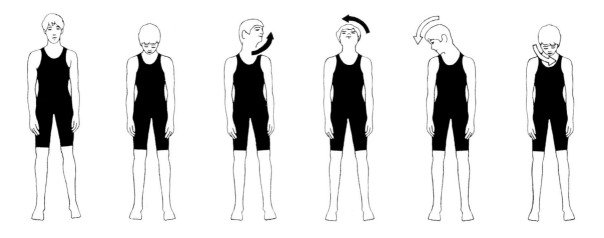

Side-to-side

Foot position 2 foot-widths

Breathing *Inhale*, left, 1 count:
Exhale, right, 1 count

Repeat ×6

Points to note Look directly ahead
and focus on an imaginary horizon
line as you rotate your head from side
to side. Keep your head and neck
upright throughout the exercise,
avoiding dipping or tilting as you reach
extreme left or right. Your torso remains
upright and relaxed, knees unlocked.
Your face is completely relaxed. Feel the
movement of the muscles at the front
and sides of the neck and also alongside
the spine down into the back.

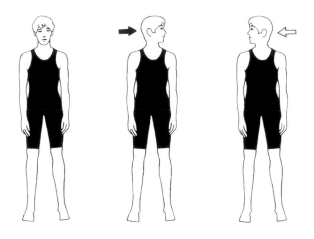

Camel

Foot position 2 foot-widths

Breathing *Inhale*, circle forward and
down, 2 counts: *Exhale*, circle back
and up, 2 counts

Repeat ×6

Points to note Keep your torso upright
and relaxed, knees unlocked. Let the
face be completely relaxed. Feel the
movement of the muscles at the front
and sides of the neck and also alongside
the spine down into the back.

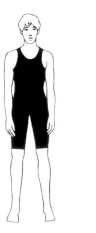
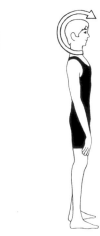

Week 4

Lung Breath

Foot position 2 foot-widths

Breathing *Inhale*, up to left, 2 counts: *Hold breath*, stretch, 2 counts: *Exhale*, down to centre, 2 counts: *Inhale*, up to right, 2 counts: *Hold breath*, stretch, 2 counts: *Exhale*, down to centre, 2 counts

Repeat ×3

Points to note Isolate the movement in your head and neck. Try to look over and down behind each shoulder to see the backs of your heels, after rotating up to each side. Feel your breath filling the top of the opposite lung.

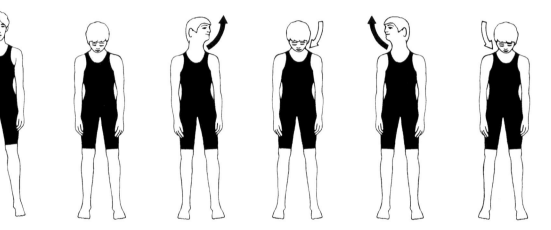

> **Week 4 Routine: Summary**
> Exercises from weeks 1–3 plus:
> Windmill ×3
> *Integration Breath ×1*
> Scythe ×6
> *Integration Breath ×1*
> Head Circles, left ×6, right ×6
> Side-to-side ×6
> Camel ×6
> Lung Breath ×3
> *Integration Breath ×1*

Cleansed, refreshed and detoxed, you are now ready to tackle your immune system and become fully resistant to disease.

WEEK 5

BOOST YOUR IMMUNE POWER

When you are younger it is easy to fool yourself into believing that all those degenerative and life-threatening diseases will only happen to other people. But are you really immune to both minor and major infections and will cancer pass you by? Are you free from allergies and do you rarely suffer from a cold? If you want to answer yes, then you're on the right track.

The concept that germs cause disease, proven by Louis Pasteur in the nine-teenth century, generated the idea that disease could be beaten and health restored by destroying the outside agent. And so we entered the era of a 'drug for a bug' – based on the approach that disease is a spanner in the works, caused by something that needs destroying, usually by drugs. While this approach has produced some very positive results, the concept of 'combat medicine' is failing to provide much-needed new breakthroughs for most of the health problems we face today. The alternative is to boost your immune system.

Think of your immune system as your own personal medical team, skilled in the art of healing, always on call, and always there to take preventative measures to avert a battle. Whether you are trying to prevent or cure an illness, your immune system is your main line of defence. It is worth looking after it so that it can serve reliably, allowing you to enjoy a happy, healthy life. Modern living, however, tends to do just the opposite – stressing, rather than strengthening, the immune army.

Week 5

ENEMIES OF THE IMMUNE SYSTEM

Smoke (tobacco and other – chimneys, incinerators, etc.)

Pollution (busy road, aeroplane flight path, industry, etc.)

Pesticides

Radiation

Carcinogenic chemicals (industrial or domestic)

Drugs (legal, illegal, medical – all requiring medical supervision for reduction or elimination, do not try it alone)

Food additives (especially colours and flavours)

Stress

Incorrect balance of food (e.g. too much salt, fat or sugar)

Accidents

Obesity or starvation

Poor mineral balance

Poor vitamin balance

Inappropriate exercise

Genetic defect

Infections (from bacteria, viruses, fungi, protozoa, worms, etc.)

Negative attitude to life

Unhappiness

Why Your Immune System Needs Boosting

Here are a few good reasons for boosting your immune system:

- Your immune system determines how fast you age.
- Your immune system fights off the viruses, bacteria and other organisms which try to attack you and cause illness, from the common ones that cause colds and thrush, to the more rare but often deadly ones like meningitis, Legionnaire's disease and AIDS.
- Your immune system has the power to destroy cancer cells as they are formed.
- Your immune system empties your body's dustbin every day, getting rid of dead cells, dead invaders, and toxic chemicals.
- Your immune system offers protection from radiation and chemical pollutants.
- Left to deteriorate, your immune system could lose control and cause allergy problems or autoimmune diseases like arthritis.
- With a struggling immune system you are ill more often, more seriously and for longer.
- With a strong immune system you are almost invincible and should be able to lead a long, healthy and active life.

CHECK YOUR IMMUNE POWER

Complete this questionnaire to find out if your immune system needs a boost.

- Do you get more than 3 colds a year?
- Do you usually get a stomach bug each year?
- Do you find it hard to shift an infection (cold or otherwise)?
- Are you prone to thrush or cystitis?
- Do you generally take at least 1 course of antibiotics each year?
- Have you had a major personal loss in the past year?
- Is there any history of cancer in your family?
- Have you ever had any growths or lumps biopsied?
- Do the glands in your neck, armpits or groin feel tender?
- Do you suffer from allergy problems?
- Do you react to insect bites with excessive swelling and redness?
- Do you have an inflammatory disease such as eczema, asthma or arthritis?
- Do you suffer from hayfever?
- Do you often have a stuffy or runny nose?
- Do you have an autoimmune disease such as rheumatoid arthritis or lupus?

- If you answer 'yes' to 7 or more questions you need to boost your immune system.
- If you answer 'yes' to between 4 and 7 questions you are beginning to show signs of low immunity and need to boost it.
- If you answer 'yes' to less than 4 questions, you are unlikely to have a problem with your immune system.
- Many people suffer from allergy of one kind or another, and now we are going to discuss them in more detail.

Week 5

Understanding and Eliminating Allergies

Allergy occurs when the body alters its normal immune response in some way, due to the presence of an allergen – a substance which brings about this immune response. The odd thing about them is that they are not always harmful in themselves; rather, it is an allergic individual who produces the wrong response.

Over the last few weeks you've been avoiding wheat and dairy products, so this week we're going to reintroduce them one by one and note whether you have any reactions to them. But first, a little more on allergies.

Who Suffers from Allergies?

Cases of allergies are rapidly increasing and are now thought to affect as many as 1 in 3 people; but it's not known whether this is due to an overall decline in our immune competence, an increased burden on our immune system, or perhaps a bit of both.

Allergies can sometimes run in families. The allergy, however, may not be the same down the generations. Allergic symptoms also change with age. A baby with eczema may grow out of it only to become an adult who suffers from hayfever.

Allergic Reactions

An allergy or sensitivity to food (and other substances) can cause or worsen a range of reactions, including:

dermatitis	behaviour problems
hives	mood changes
eczema	alcoholism
migraine	fits
hayfever	heart problems
asthma	inflammatory bowel diseases
water retention	arthritis

Allergic symptoms may also affect other areas of the body, such as the hands, stomach, feet, throat, blood vessels and bladder – in fact, almost anywhere. With most allergic problems, it is a question of trying to find the triggers that bring about the condition.

Testing for Allergies

Testing for allergy is notoriously difficult. There are numerous tests available, each claiming to be accurate, but trials have shown that such tests can produce widely varying results. Some are, however, reasonably accurate, especially in detecting particular types of allergies. When you are testing for allergies, it is important to avoid alcohol, as it could interfere with the results by affecting the integrity of the gut.

Avoidance Testing

Perhaps one of the most accurate methods for discovering food allergens is to avoid suspect foods for a time and then watch for any reaction when they are reintroduced into the diet. Foods that provoke an immediate response (peanuts or seafood for example) may have to be avoided for life. Others that produce a more delayed reaction may be reduced or avoided for some time. It is generally recommended to avoid suspect foods for at least 3 months, then test again. After long-term avoidance (up to 6 months) it is unlikely that any 'memory' of a reaction to that food will remain. Another option, after a strict 1-month avoidance, is to 'rotate' foods so a sensitive food is only eaten every 4 days to reduce the build-up of allergen–antibody complexes.

Reintroduction Plan

This week it's time to check whether you have any reactions to wheat or dairy produce. To do this, eat something containing these foods – wait 3 days between introducing each substance – and note anything you feel, e.g. bloating, indigestion, constipation, tiredness, water retention, irritability, grogginess or whatever. Remember that you may not experience a reaction immediately, it could show up the next day – so it is important to wait 3 days before you

Week 5

try the next food in order to be able to detect which food it is that is causing a reaction, if any.

	Introduce	Reaction over next 48 hours
DAY 1	wheat bread, crackers, pasta, noodles	
DAY 4	dairy produce milk, cheese	

If you do have a reaction to any of the foods, it's probably best that you stay off them for another 4 weeks, then have them only once every 4 days, if that. Many people who find they react to such foods, even only mildly, avoid them most of the time.

Immune-boosting Nutrients

These nutrients perform a vital role in helping our immune system to cope with the daily attacks on it.

Vitamin A

This is responsible for maintaining an active thymus – the master gland of the immune system. Vitamin A is a powerful antiviral vitamin, mainly because its inclusion in cell membranes makes them stronger and more resistant to viral attack. It is particularly important for areas with a high risk of infection, such as the respiratory system, the gut and the genito-urinary tract.

B Complex

This family of essential nutrients is important for every single cell of the body, including those of the immune system. Folic acid and pyridoxine (B6) probably have the most effect on the immune function. It has been found that a baby's thymus is larger and its immune system stronger if the mother has had a good supply of folic acid, choline, B12 and methionine. A B6 deficiency causes a decrease in the activity of the phagocytic cells so that we cannot clean up inside as effectively as we should. Phagocytes get rid of 'invaders', dead cells and any other unwanted matter.

Vitamin C

In truth a whole book could be written about vitamin C and its effects on the immune system. There is no question that more vitamin C means better immune function. Here are some of its key roles in boosting your immunity:

- Vitamin C is strongly antiviral and has proved successful against every virus tested so far, from HIV to the common cold.
- Vitamin C can be bacteriostatic or bactericidal i.e. it can hinder the growth of bacteria or kill them, depending on the bug.
- Vitamin C also helps sore eyes and runny nose, as it is a natural antihistamine.

Most animals are able to make vitamin C in the body from glucose. Humans, other primates, guinea pigs, the Indian fruit-eating bat and the red-vented bulbul bird do not. All these rely on vitamin C in their diet and would die of scurvy without it.

Vitamin E

Vitamin E is necessary for a normal antibody response and works with other nutrients to improve our resistance to infection. It is very effective in protecting us from air pollution, particularly that due to exhausts, air purifiers or deodorisers which generate ozone.

Calcium and Magnesium

The mineral calcium is vital for the immune system. It is needed by all phagocytic cells in order to attach to and ingest foreign material. It is needed to destroy viruses and for fever production, which enhances the role of immune cells. Calcium works with magnesium, which is no less important for immunity: it is vital for antibody production, the thymus and much more. Deficiency can cause a rise in histamine levels and hence increase allergic reactions.

Iron

Iron is essential for the production of antibodies, white blood cells and enzymes made by immune cells. However, bacteria need iron for reproduction, so it is wise to avoid iron in supplements or iron-rich foods when suffering from a bacterial infection.

Week 5

Selenium

Research on animals has shown that there is no antibody production at all when they are deprived of vitamin E and selenium. White blood cells also lose their efficiency in recognising invaders without it. Deficiency is associated with cancer. British soil is very low in selenium, so food grown in it is too; Britain has one of the highest cancer rates.

Zinc

Zinc is a very versatile mineral, involved in over 200 of the body's known enzymes, and it is crucial for immune health. Deficiency causes shrinking of the thymus – the master immune gland. It is also needed to produce enzymes needed for the elimination of routinely produced cancer cells (not for the large amounts once cancer is established). The mineral zinc has also proved to be anti-viral and is available in lozenges for coughs and colds. There is a high level of zinc in seminal fluid, so men with high sexual activity need more zinc.

ZINC CHECK

Do you suffer from:

- poor sense of taste or smell?
- white marks on fingernails?
- frequent infections?
- stretch marks?
- acne or greasy skin?
- low fertility?
- pale skin?
- tendency to depression?
- loss of appetite?

If you have 4 or more of these symptoms, you are probably low in zinc. Main food sources are meat, shellfish, eggs. Seeds, especially pumpkin, are probably the best source.

Fighting Infections Naturally

Lying on his deathbed, Louis Pasteur stated, 'the host is more important than the invader'. It's increasingly being recognised that we are more likely to succumb to bugs if we are run down, confirming the adage: 'Prevention is better than cure.' The best line of defence is to keep the immune system strong for when the next invader comes along. We are all exposed to germs that cause infectious diseases, but those of us with strong immune systems fight back more effectively and either avoid symptoms of the illness entirely or have a milder attack.

Immune cells work better in a warmer environment, which is why the body 'gets a temperature' when you are ill. Keep your room warm, and get some sleep. Sleep is the time when you heal, repair and produce chemicals which stimulate the immune system. Eliminate other energy-robbers such as alcohol, smoke, strong light, loud sounds, over-eating, highly processed foods, stress, sex and over-exertion. Drink lots of water to dilute and eliminate toxins produced during the battle and to prevent dehydration. Avoid salt, fatty foods and those which are mucous-forming (dairy produce, eggs and meat). Also avoid concentrated protein foods if you have any sort of stomach upset.

A–Z of Natural Remedies for Boosting the Immune System

A – vitamin A is one of the key immune-boosting nutrients. It helps strengthen the skin, inside and out, and therefore acts in the first line of defence, keeping the lungs, digestive tract and skin intact. By strengthening cell membranes, it keep viruses out.

Aloe vera has immune-boosting, antiviral and antiseptic properties, probably due to its high concentration of mucopolysaccharides. It's a good all-round tonic, as well as a booster during any infection.

Antioxidants are substances that detoxify 'free radicals'. These include vitamins A, C, E, beta-carotene, zinc, selenium and many other non-essential substances from silymarin (milk thistle), pycnogenol, lipoic acid, bioflavonoids and bilberry extract.

Artemisia is a natural antifungal, antiparasitic and antibacterial agent.

Bee pollen is a natural antibiotic. It's probably best as a general tonic. Quality varies considerably, so pick your source carefully. Be careful if you're pollen-sensitive or allergic to bee-stings.

Beta-carotene is the vegetable source of pre-vitamin A and an antioxidant in its own right. Carrot or watermelon juice is a great way to take this all-round infection fighter.

C – vitamin C is an incredible antiviral agent.

Cat's claw (*Uncaria tomentosa*) is a powerful antiviral, antioxidant and immune boosting agent from the Peruvian rain forest plant. It is available as a tea or in supplements. The tea tastes good with added blackcurrant concentrate.

E – vitamin E is the most important fat-soluble antioxidant. So it protects essential fats in nuts and seeds from going rancid.

Echinacea is a great 'all-rounder' with antiviral and antibacterial properties. It's the original Red Indian 'snakeroot'.

Garlic contains allicin, which is antiviral, antifungal and antibacterial. Rich in sulphur-containing amino acids, it also acts as an antioxidant. It's undoubtedly an important ally in fighting infections, and garlic-eaters have the lowest incidence of cancer. Consider a clove or capsule equivalent daily.

Ginger is particularly good for sore throats and stomach upsets. Put 6 slices of fresh ginger in a thermos with a stick of cinnamon and boiling water, and 5 minutes later you have a delicious, soothing tea. You can add a little lemon and honey too.

Grapefruit seed extract, also called Citricidal, is a powerful antibiotic, anti-fungal and antiviral agent. The great advantage, however, is that it doesn't adversely effect beneficial gut bacteria. It comes in drops and can be swallowed, gargled with or used as nose drops or ear drops, depending on the site of infection.

Lysine is an amino acid that helps get rid of the herpes virus. During an infection its best to limit arginine-rich foods such as beans, lentils, nuts and chocolate and take a lysine supplement plus vitamin C.

Mushrooms such as shiitake, maiitake, reishi or ganoderma, traditionally believed by Chinese Taoists to confer immortality, have all been shown to contain immune-boosting polysaccharides.

Probiotics, as opposed to antibiotics, are beneficial bacteria that promote health and are available in capsule or powder form. They are best used to restore balance in the digestive tract, for example during a stomach bug.

Selenium is an immune-enhancing mineral that also acts as an antioxidant.

Week 5

Tea tree oil is an Australian remedy with antiseptic and antifungal properties. Great for rubbing on the chest or gargling (diluted), in the bath, or steam inhaling, and also helps keep mosquitoes away.

Zinc is the most important immune-boosting mineral, well worth upping during any infection. There's no question it helps fight infections. For sore throats, zinc lozenges are also available.

---

7 Ways to Stop a Cold Dead in its Tracks

1. Take 3 grams of vitamin C immediately and then 2g every 4 hours (or 3 times a day) until symptoms subside. Alternatively, mix 6 grams of vitamin C powder in fruit juice diluted with water and drink throughout the day. Some people prefer calcium ascorbate, a less acidic form of vitamin C.

2. Supplement other immune-boosting nutrients, especially vitamins A and E, selenium and zinc.

3. Eat lightly, preferably relying mainly on fruits and vegetables, including foods rich in vitamins A and C, for example, carrot, beetroot, green peppers and citrus fruit. Avoid mucous-forming and fatty foods, i.e. meat, eggs and milk products. These make your lymph limp — and lymphatic fluid is the main transport system for immune cells which carry invading viruses to lymph nodes for further punishment.

4. Avoid all alcohol, cigarettes, tea and coffee. Drink plenty of water and herb teas.

5. Boost your immunity with herbs. Drink 2 cups of cat's claw tea a day, have 15 drops of echinacea tincture twice a day and, if you have flu or a severe cold, also have a dessertspoon of Sambucol (elderberry extract) 4 times a day.

6. Take it easy. Do everything slowly and avoid stress. Get some rest and plenty of sleep.

7. If you think you've won the battle, wait at least 24 hours before reducing the vitamins down to 1 gram of vitamin C 3 times a day, and one immune-boosting vitamin and mineral supplement in the morning. Once you have been well for 3 days go back to your normal supplement programme.

Week 5

Immune-boosting Teas

Pour freshly boiled water over any of the following teas, allow to steep for 5 minutes (ideally in a Thermos flask), and you've got a delicious cup of soothing, refreshing tea . . .

- Cat's claw tea with a dash of sugar-free blackcurrant cordial.
- Freshly grated ginger with cinnamon sticks.
- Freshly grated ginger with lemon juice and honey.
- Fresh lime juice.
- Cinnamon sticks, cloves, cardamom pods and sliced ginger.

IMMUNE-BOOSTING Action Plan

DOs

- Drink cat's claw tea daily.

- Introduce wheat and dairy produce as explained on page 130.

- Eat plenty of colourful, varied fresh fruit and vegetables, especially those that are red, orange and purple, such as berries, sweet potatoes and red peppers.

- Eat plenty of seeds such as pumpkin and sunflower as snacks, in salads, on cereal, etc.

- Include plenty of vitamin C-rich foods in your diet – peppers, broccoli, peas, cabbage, lemons, oranges, strawberries.

And as always . . .

1 heaped tablespoon of ground seeds or 1 tablespoon of cold-pressed seed oil.

2 servings of beans, lentils, quinoa, tofu (soya), or 'seed' vegetables.

3 pieces of fresh fruit such as apples, pears, bananas, berries, melon or citrus fruit.

4 servings of wholegrains such as rice, millet, rye, oats, corn or quinoa.

5 servings of dark green, leafy and root vegetables such as watercress, carrots, sweet potatoes, broccoli, spinach, green beans, peas and peppers.

6 glasses of water, diluted juices, herb or fruit teas.

7 Eat whole, organic, raw food as much as you can.

8 Avoid any form of sugar, white, refined or processed food with chemical additives.

9 Avoid all stimulants – coffee, tea, cigarettes.

10 Relax during your meal and chew your food well.

DON'Ts

■ Avoid alcohol completely.

IMMUNE-BOOSTING Menus

Below are some meal recommendations for Week 5. You can of course use or adapt recipes from other weeks which comply to the current 'Dos and Don'ts'.

Breakfast
Choose from:
- Ultimate Power Breakfast (page 174)
- Get Up & Go (page 213) blended with skimmed or soya milk and a banana
- Healthy Scrambled Eggs (page 178)
- Oat Porridge (page 176)

Other recipes can be taken from *The Optimum Nutrition Cookbook* (Piatkus, 1999), which I co-authored with Judy Ridgway.

Lunch
Choose from:
- Provençal Tuna Salad in a Bun (page 184)
- Bulgarian Salad with Feta Cheese (page 189)
- Sweet Potato and Carrot Soup (page 184)

Other recommended recipes, taken from *The Optimum Nutrition Cookbook*, include: Rye Deckers with Avocado, Smoked Chicken and Cranberry Sauce; Spicy Red Bean Dip Sandwich; Quick Salmon Pâté; Hummus, Cucumber and Alfalfa Sprouts on Rye Crispbread.

Week 5

Dinner

Choose from:

- Duck Slivers with Orange Beansprouts and Chinese Egg Noodles (page 201)
- Vegetable Parcels with Chilli Sauce and Kiwi Salsa (page 210)
- Roasted Red Peppers with Goat's Cheese and Sweet Potato Mash (page 202)

Other recommended recipes, taken from *The Optimum Nutrition Cookbook*, include: Stuffed Squash with Watercress Salad; Salmon Tarragon Fishcakes with Tomato Sauce on a Bed of Spinach; Mexican Spinach with Baked Yams; Chickpea Crumble with Leafy Avocado Salad.

IMMUNE-BOOSTING Supplements

As always	Breakfast	Lunch	Dinner
Multi-vitamin/mineral	2		
Vitamin C 1,000mg	1		
Antioxidant complex	2		

Add			
Vitamin C 1,000mg	1		

Optional

- If you have a cold or are run down, take zinc, echinacea and cat's claw.

Optional to continue	Breakfast	Lunch	Dinner
Chromium 200mcg	1		
Digestive enzymes	1	1	1
Herbal Aloe Detox	1 tablespoon	1 tablespoon	
Essential Balance	1 tablespoon		

IMMUNE-BOOSTING Awareness Exercise

The lymphatic system is vital for super immunity. Immune cells are transported along lymphatic vessels, while invading organisms and misbehaving cells are taken to lymph nodes for destruction. Their remains are eliminated via the lymphatic system, which drains into the digestive tract and the skin. You can

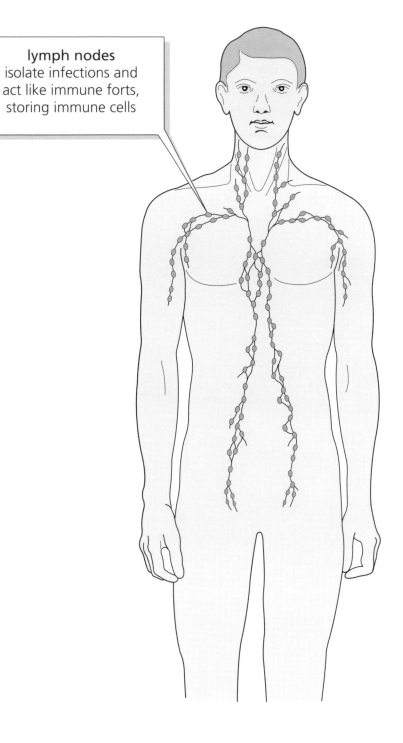

lymph nodes
isolate infections and
act like immune forts,
storing immune cells

Lymphatic system

improve your immune strength by stimulating the lymphatic system and promoting lymphatic drainage.

- **Have a shower or bath every day** and vigorously brush your skin with either a skin brush, a loofah or a buffing cloth.

- **Wake up your lymphatic nodes with cold water.** At the end of your bath or shower turn the water to cold and have a brief cold shower. Pay particular attention to the three areas of the body that concentrate lymph nodes – the neck, the armpits and groin. If you do not have a shower, splash these areas with cold water.

- **Be aware of the early warning signs of immune invasion** (see page 127), especially the following:

Tender glands in the neck, armpits or groin
Bloodshot or itchy eyes
Sore throat
Blocked nose or excessive mucus
Feeling tired or sleepy
Feeling unusually cold or hot and sweaty

If you have a number of these possible indicators of infection consider the following courses of action:

- Increase your intake of vitamin C to 1–3 grams every 4 hours.
- Supplement more zinc, echinacea and cat's claw *or*
- Drink cat's claw tea 2–3 times a day.
- Take it easy until you regain your resilience.

WEEK 5 Psychocalisthenics Exercises

Here are 4 new *Psychocalisthenics* exercises for Week 5.

Candle/Plough

Lower yourself to the floor and lie down on your back

Breathing *Inhale*, up to Candle, 6 counts: *Exhale*, hold Candle, 6 counts:
Inhale, over to Plough, 6 counts: *Exhale*, hold Plough, 6 counts:
Inhale, back up to Candle, 6 counts:
Exhale, hold Candle, 6 counts:
Inhale, down to floor, 6 counts:
Exhale, relax, 6 counts

Repeat ×3

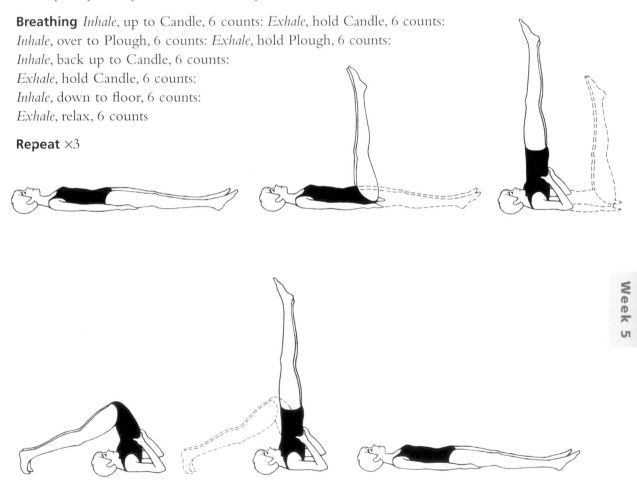

Points to note Concentrate on keeping your legs straight at the knee as you bring them up to 90 degrees to the torso, using the abdominal muscles. Continue on up, supporting your back with your hands as close to your shoulder blades as possible. Relax your face and jaw. Check that your weight is on your elbows as much as on your shoulders and neck. Maintain this distribution of weight as you bring your legs, knees straight, over behind your head, until your toes touch the floor, or as far as possible. Try shifting your hips to bring your weight more on to your elbows. Be gentle. Feel the stretch from the toes all the way to the base of your skull. As you bring your legs back up to the vertical position and then back down to the floor, feel your abdominal and groin muscles working. As you lower your feet, move your arms to your sides, palms down, to steady yourself. Keep your arms, wrists and hands flat on the floor. Relax your shoulders and neck so your head does not come up as your legs descend and your spine curls on to the floor.

Bow

Breathing *Inhale*, up, 2 counts: *Exhale*, down, 2 counts

Repeat ×6

Points to note The legs are straight and the fingers point toward the toes. Look above your feet, for a straight back and neck and better balance. Start with your arms at your sides, palms down. The arms return to this position at the end of each Bow. Make two quick full inhalations as you come up into the Bow, and two quick full exhalations as you relax the Bow and come down to the floor. The breathing makes the movement.

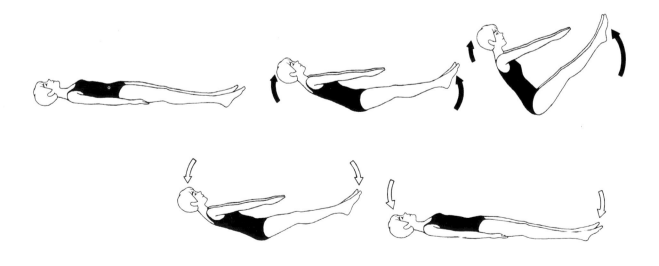

Leg Circles

Breathing *Inhale*, circle up, out and around, 6 counts: *Exhale*, circle down, out and around, 6 counts

Repeats ×6

Points to note Focus on your breathing throughout this exercise, making the inhale and exhale sound loud and clear. Your legs are straight. Keep your hips in contact with the floor, or with your hands palms down on the floor slightly under your hips, so that you are getting maximum stretch in the hamstring muscles as your legs make the circles. Your feet do not come down to the floor between each circle, thus strongly working your belly and thigh muscles. Match your breath with the movement, seeing that the breath is guiding you through the rotations.

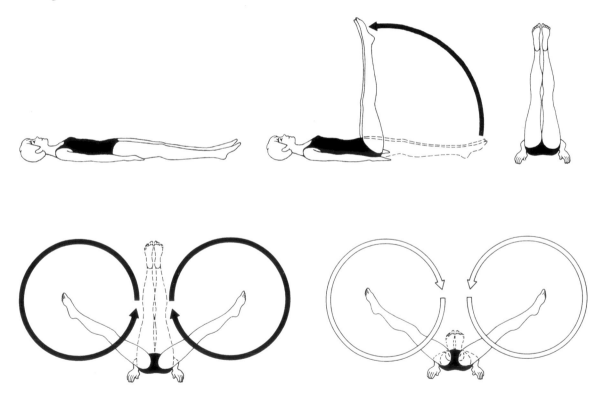

Scissors

Breathing *Inhale*, open, 1 count: *Exhale*, cross, 1 count

Repeat ×6 alternating left over right/right over left

Points to note Raise your feet 30cm above the ground. With the feet and legs at the correct height, your abdominal muscles are getting a better stretch. Keep your legs straight at the knees so that they are like the blades of a pair of scissors, sharply crisscrossing rather than waving about in the air. Keep your head resting on the ground throughout.

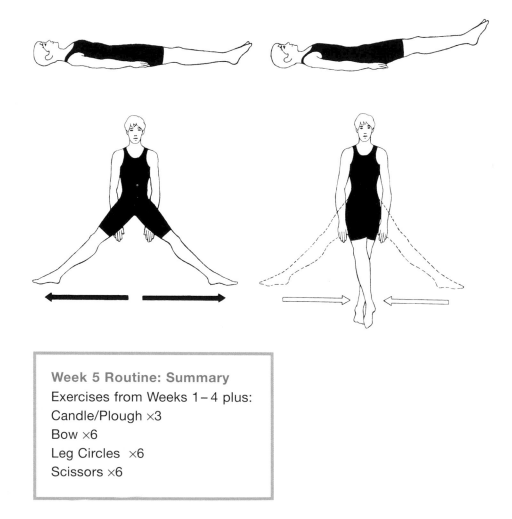

Week 5 Routine: Summary
Exercises from Weeks 1–4 plus:
Candle/Plough ×3
Bow ×6
Leg Circles ×6
Scissors ×6

You only have one week to go before completing the superhealth programme. You are well on your way to becoming fit and healthy.

IMPROVE YOUR MEMORY AND MOOD

Your intelligence and memory aren't purely determined by your genetic programming – although there is clearly an in-built element to them both. The development of learning skills and what you eat do make a big difference to your mental abilities.

The brain and nervous system – our mental 'hardware' – are made up of a network of 'neurons', special cells which are each capable of forming tens of thousands of connections with others. Thinking is thought to represent a pattern of activity across this network. Such activity, or signals, involves neurotransmitters, the chemical messengers in the brain. When we learn, we actually programme the wiring of the brain. When we think, we change the activity of neurotransmitters. Since both the brain and neurotransmitters are derived from nutrients in food, it is logical to think that what you eat has a bearing on your mental performance.

Balancing Blood Sugar

Keeping your blood sugar balanced is probably the most important factor in maintaining an even energy, mood and concentration as well as many other factors including weight. When the level of glucose in your blood drops you are likely to experience a whole host of symptoms including fatigue, poor concentration, irritability, nervousness, depression, excessive thirst, sweating, headaches and digestive problems. You are likely to want to eat or drink something – starchy, sweet, coffee or tea – to give you a lift. The glucose in your bloodstream is available to body cells for them to make energy. An estimated 3 in every 10 people have a compromised ability to keep an even blood sugar level – it may go too high and then drop too low. The result, over the years, is that they become increasingly lethargic and fat. On the other hand, if you can control your blood sugar levels, you are likely to have more constant energy as well as balanced moods and concentration. More on this subject was covered in Week 1 of your 6 Weeks to Superhealth programme.

Brain Fats

ARE YOU DEFICIENT IN ESSENTIAL FATS?

C T

- dry skin, eczema or dry eyes ☑ Y
- dry hair or dandruff ☐
- inflammatory health problems
  e.g. arthritis ☐
- excessive thirst or sweating ☐
- PMS or breast pain ☐
- water retention ☐

C T

- frequent infections ☐
- poor memory ☐
- learning difficulties ☐
- irritability ☐
- hyperactivity ☐
- high blood pressure or high
  blood fats ☐

If you answered yes to 6 or more, you probably need to increase your intake of essential fats.

Conclusive research now clearly shows that the amount and type of fat consumed during foetal development, infancy, childhood, adolescence, adulthood, old age and indeed every day of our life has a profound effect on how we think and feel. The brain and nervous system are dependent on a balance of fats.

Every nerve cell in the brain is surrounded by a membrane composed of fatty molecules. The myelin sheath, which adds an additional layer of insulation to many of these nerve cells, is roughly 75 per cent fat (one-quarter of which is cholesterol). Disturbance in myelination, such as in the disease multiple sclerosis, has profound effects on health, especially if it occurs during critical periods of brain development.

The making of intelligence involves the careful connecting of billions of developing nerve cells; each one connects to up to 20,000 others, many requiring myelination. The connection points are called synapses, across which neurotransmitter chemicals, which facilitate the transport of nerve signals, travel and dock into receptor sites. These receptor sites are embedded in the myelin, which is made out of molecules which contain fats. It is the balance of the fats which appears to be critical for the brain's structure and function. So for brain health both Omega 3 and Omega 6 fats must be present in your diet.

Omega 3 Fats

While essential fats are needed for both the structure and the function of the brain and nervous system, they can also be converted into messenger molecules called prostaglandins which affect the release of neurotransmitters and hence the transmission of nerve impulses. The prostaglandins derived from Omega 3 fats (see page 95) are essential for proper brain function, affecting vision, learning ability, co-ordination and mood as well as countless other body functions.

In fact, the level of the Omega 3 fats, DHA and EPA – both found in fish oils – are markers for intelligence. Studies have found that the blood levels of these essential fats correlate with intellectual performance and learning ability at the age of 5. The World Health Organisation now recommends that baby formula feeds include these oils.

The best seed oils for Omega 3 fats are flax (also known as linseed), hemp and pumpkin. In much the same way as evening primrose oil bypasses the first 'conversion' stage of linoleic acid, eating carnivorous fish or their oils bypasses the first two conversion stages of alpha-linolenic acid, to provide EPA and DHA. This is why fish-eaters like the Japanese have 3 times the Omega 3 fats in their body fat of the average American. Vegans, who eat more seeds and nuts, have twice the Omega 3 fat level in their body fat of the average American.

Omega 6 Fats

Omega 6 fats (see page 96) are also essential for mental health. Of all the tissues of the body, the brain has the highest proportion of Omega 6 fats. They are part

Week 6

of nerve tissue and influence brain function. Numerous studies have shown that schizophrenics have low levels. A survey by the World Health Organisation found that the countries which had the most severe schizophrenia were those whose intake of essential fats was lowest.

Adding evening primrose oil to the diet of alcoholics going through withdrawal has been shown to dramatically reduce symptoms, and, in the long term, improves memory. Due to its reported effects on memory, evening primrose oil was given to Alzheimer's patients in a controlled trial. Once again, highly significant improvements in memory and mental function were found.

This family of fats comes exclusively from seeds and their oils. The best seed oils are hemp, pumpkin, sunflower, safflower, sesame, corn, walnut, soybean and wheatgerm oil. About half of the fats in these oils comes from the Omega 6 family, mainly as linoleic acid.

CHECK YOUR MEMORY AND MOOD

- Is your memory deteriorating?
- Do you find it hard to concentrate and often get confused?
- Are you often depressed?
- Do you become anxious easily or wake up with a feeling of anxiety?
- Does stress leave you feeling exhausted?
- Do you have mood swings and become angry or irritable easily?
- Are you lacking in motivation?
- Do you sometimes feel like you're going crazy?
- Do you have misperceptions where things don't look or sound right or you feel distant or disconnected?
- Do you suffer from insomnia?
- Does your mind ever go blank?
- Do you often find you can remember things from the past but forget what you did yesterday?
- Do you wake up in the early hours of the morning?

- Are you prone to premenstrual tension?

- Is your mood noticeably worse in the winter?

- If you answer 'yes' to 7 or more questions, it is likely that your memory and/or mood need support from dietary changes and supplements.

- If you answer 'yes' to between 4 and 7 questions, you are beginning to show signs of mood/memory difficulties.

- If you answer 'yes' to fewer than 4 questions, you are unlikely to have memory and/or mood problems.

- If you recognise some or all of these symptoms, you are probably in need of some memory-enhancing nutrients.

Nutrients and Mood

Every one of the 50 known essential nutrients, with the exception of vitamin D, has a role to play in promoting brain function. For more general information on vitamins, see Part 2.

B Vitamins

The B complex group of vitamins are vital for mental health. Deficiency of any one of the 8 B vitamins will rapidly affect how you think and feel. This is because they are water-soluble and rapidly pass out of the body so we need a regular intake throughout the day. Also, since the brain uses a very large amount of these nutrients, a short-term deficiency will affect mental abilities.

B vitamins have many roles to play in ensuring optimal brain function. Niacin, or B3, is particularly good for memory enhancement. In one study 141mg of niacin was given daily to a group of subjects of various ages. Memory was improved by 10–40 per cent in all age groups.

B5 (pantothenic acid) has many functions in the body. It is essential for the brain and helps improve energy. It is essential for the formation of acetylcholine (see page 152). B12 has been shown in laboratory experiments to accelerate the rate that rats learn – it is very important for the health of nerve cells.

B6 (pyridoxine) has an important role in brain function as it is essential for the manufacture of neurotransmitters. It is also necessary for the conversion of

Week 6

amino acids into serotonin – a deficiency in this important neurotransmitter can cause depression and other problems. See the section on 5-HTP for more information on serotonin (page 154). One study showed that about a fifth of depressed people who took part were deficient in pyridoxine.

It is important to remember that B vitamins should be taken in a complex, i.e. all together, and if you wish to concentrate on a specific B vitamin take this in conjunction with a lower-dose complex.

Vitamin C

Vitamin C does more than stop you getting colds. It has many roles to play in the brain, helping to balance neurotransmitters. While not so spectacular as niacin, vitamin C has been shown to reduce the symptoms of schizophrenia.

Calcium and Magnesium – Natural Tranquillisers

'My nerves are shot to pieces' is how many people instinctively describe their state when feeling anxious, edgy and unable to relax. Our nerves send messages through a series of chemicals, which change the positive or negative charge of our nerve cells. This difference in charge creates a current of electricity, passing on the nervous signal. Just like an out-of-tune car, these signals can get out of synch. Calcium collects inside and outside the cell, to help turn on a signal, while magnesium acts to relax the cell signal – so a lack of magnesium helps create that edgy feeling.

Next time you reach for a sleeping pill reach for calcium and magnesium instead. As a natural sleeping aid 600mg of calcium and 400mg of magnesium usually does the trick.

Magnesium has many roles to play in the nervous system, and the possibility of magnesium deficiency being a cause of mental problems is starting to be researched more thoroughly. Magnesium is perhaps the second most commonly deficient mineral. Without it it's easy to become 'wound up', anxious, hyperactive and irritable.

Manganese – the Forgotten Mineral

Too much or too little manganese affects the way our brain functions. An excess, found occasionally in miners inhaling dust from manganese ore, results in psychosis and nervous disorders similar to Parkinson's disease. However, excess is rare since manganese is both hard to absorb and is readily excreted. Too little manganese is associated with insomnia, restlessness, non-productive activity and elevated blood pressure.

Zinc – the Mental Element

Zinc is perhaps the most commonly deficient mineral, and the most critical nutrient for mental health. The average intake in Britain is 7.5mg, which is half the RDA of 15mg. This means that half the British population get less than half the level of zinc thought to protect against deficiency. Zinc deficiency is associated with schizophrenia, depression, anxiety, anorexia, delinquency, hyperactivity, autism – in short, almost all types of mental health problem.

Memory Enhancers

How Good is Your Memory?

Try this simple short-term memory test, based on your ability to remember random numbers. Each line contains 12 random numbers. Have someone read you any one of these lines, allowing about one second for each number, announcing each number clearly in a monotonous voice.

1	5	2	7	4	0	8	1	7	2	6	3
3	6	8	2	4	5	7	1	2	9	4	6
4	2	0	8	5	1	2	0	7	6	3	4
9	9	3	8	7	9	5	4	6	7	5	2
2	8	2	1	5	8	3	0	5	9	2	8
5	4	5	6	9	8	2	5	7	0	3	5
1	5	8	0	1	9	7	6	5	8	2	4
0	2	5	8	7	5	3	6	9	5	1	9
6	0	7	3	9	1	4	6	8	2	7	2
3	6	8	4	2	5	9	7	1	3	3	5
4	0	2	8	5	6	5	4	7	8	3	8
8	3	6	4	5	8	2	6	7	1	2	6

How many numbers can you recall, in the right sequence? If you can get the first 6 right you score 6 points. Try this 3 times. You should find you have an 'average' digit recall score. Try this test again in a month to see how much your short-term memory improves as you attain higher and higher levels of superhealth.

Although studies have yet to be performed to show it, there is no good reason to assume that adults can't achieve similar benefits in sharpening intelligence through optimum nutrition. But what about sharpening your memory? What about the milder and more commonly experienced memory decline that we tend to ascribe to the normal process of ageing or simply to personality differences? Is there room for improvement here?

According to the drug companies, there is. 'Age-associated memory impairment affects many more people than Alzheimer's disease, although, it's certainly true, it is a much less severe condition. We believe at least 4 million people in the UK suffer from this,' says Dr Paul Williams from Glaxo Pharmaceuticals, who have been developing drugs to enhance memory and mental performance.

For the pharmaceutical industry, the advantage of these drugs is that they are not nutrients but man-made substances, i.e. they can be patented after millions of pounds have been spent on research. The disadvantage of such man-made chemicals is that, although modelled on nutrients, they are alien to the human body. Of course, with most of these new smart drugs, the long-term effects have yet to be discovered.

There is an alternative and safer way to enhance your memory, mind and mood – that is to ensure you are taking in optimal levels of the nutrients from which your body can make key brain chemicals, through your diet and in supplements.

Choline and DMAE

Perhaps the key brain chemical for memory is acetylcholine, a neurotransmitter that is derived from the nutrient choline. Fish, especially sardines, are rich in choline, hence the old wives' tale of fish being good for the brain. Acetylcholine is partly responsible for how we connect sensory information with memories and then respond appropriately. However, you don't simply make more acetylcholine by eating choline; vitamin B5 is essential for the formation of acetylcholine in the body. Some forms of choline cross more easily from the blood into the brain – such as phosphatidyl choline and a precursor (a substance which can be converted) for choline called DMAE (short for dimethylaminoethanol) which accelerates the brain's production of acetylcholine.

While both of these substances can be made by the brain and are therefore not classified as essential nutrients, there is evidence that supplementing has positive effects on memory and learning. Slight chemical variations of DMAE have been marketed as the drug Deaner or Deanol, which has proven highly effective in helping those with learning problems, attention deficit disorder, memory and behaviour problems. DMAE is also found naturally in fish.

Pyroglutamate

Another key brain chemical that appears to enhance memory and mental function is the amino acid pyroglutamate and its derivatives, which are highly concentrated in the human brain and spinal fluid. In fact, so powerful are its effects that there are now many slight variations of this key brain chemical being marketed as drugs for learning and memory-related problems such as Alzheimer's. Numerous studies using these 'smart drugs' have proven to enhance memory and mental function, not only in those with pronounced memory decline but also in people with so-called normal memory function.

Phosphatidyl Serine

Known as the memory molecule, phosphatidyl serine (PS) is another smart nutrient that can genuinely boost your brain power. PS is a type of phospholipid – these substances are essential for the health of the liver, immune system, nerves and brain. PS is especially plentiful in the brain and is the subject of an increasing amount of scientific evidence that supplements improve memory, mood, stress resistance, learning and concentration.

While the body can make its own PS, we rely on receiving some directly from diet, which makes PS a semi-essential nutrient. The trouble is that modern diets are deficient in PS unless you happen to eat a lot of organ meats, in which case you may take in 50mg a day. A vegetarian diet is unlikely to achieve even 10mg a day. The secret to the memory-boosting properties of PS is probably due to its ability to help brain cells communicate. Unlike neurotransmitters, which are messenger molecules which deliver messages from one neuron to another, phosphatidyl serine is a vital part of the structure of the 'docking port' for these messenger molecules, technically known as the receptor site.

Ginkgo Biloba

Ginkgo biloba is a herbal remedy that has been used for memory enhancement in the East for thousands of years. It comes from one of the oldest species of tree known. Research has shown that it improves short-term and age-related memory loss, slow thinking, depression, circulation and blood flow to the brain. It has also been seen to significantly improve Parkinson's and Alzheimer's disease in one year.

Ginkgo usually comes in capsule form and you should look for a brand that shows the flavonoid concentration, which determines strength. The recommended flavonoid concentration is 24 per cent, of which one would take

120–160mg in 2–3 divided doses. It is suggested that you try the product for between 3 and 6 months before evaluating the results.

A number of supplement companies produce 'smart nutrient' formulae that contain a combination of these memory enhancers.

Mood Enhancers

5-HTP – Nature's Blues Buster

While many of the nutrients discussed above will improve your memory and mental function, they will also help stabilise your mood. If you're feeling depressed, you may be deficient in serotonin, a vital brain chemical that helps to keep you in a good mood. It is thought that possibly half of all people with clinical depression have serotonin deficiency, which is much more common in women. The connection between a deficiency of the neurotransmitter serotonin and mood is now undisputed. We all produce some serotonin, but many people who are depressed produce too little. Indeed, many people do respond to drugs such as the ubiquitous Prozac which increase the amount of serotonin in circulation in the body. The trouble is that these kinds of drugs induce unpleasant side-effects in about a quarter of those who take them and severe reactions in a minority. Due to the long list of complications – from constipation to convulsions – demand is high for a safer, natural alternative. Scientific evidence overwhelmingly backs the use of 5-HTP.

■ **What is 5-HTP?** 5-HTP, or 5-hydroxytryptophan, is a substance extracted from a shrubby African plant called griffonia (*Griffonia simplicifolia*), grown mostly in Ghana and the Ivory Coast. Each seed contains between 5 and 10 per cent 5-HTP. It is a precursor to the neurotransmitter serotonin, i.e. it can be converted to serotonin in the body. Neurotransmitters are chemical messengers made in the body which help nerve cells fire messages from one to the next.

Scientific research shows that there are few adverse effects associated with the use of 5-HTP, although some people do experience mild digestive disturbances such as nausea when taking higher doses.

■ **How Does 5-HTP work?** To understand the role that 5-HTP plays in increasing serotonin levels, first you need to know a little about serotonin production in the body. Through a set of chemical reactions involving various enzymes which are in turn dependent on certain nutrients, the body can convert the amino acid (protein constituent) tryptophan, which is present in many foods, to 5-HTP, and from there to serotonin. So, put simply, 5-HTP provides the brain with the raw material to make serotonin. Studies have proven that this nutrient is as effective as the best anti-depressants without the side-effects.

Tryptophan, however, can also shoot off down various other metabolic pathways to make other substances once it is in the body, so a more reliable way of ensuring that serotonin is increased is to take 5-HTP itself.

The conversion of 5-HTP to serotonin relies on an enzyme called 5-HTP carboxylase, which, in order to function optimally itself, requires adequate amounts of the co-factor nutrients: vitamins B6 and biotin and the mineral zinc. So, it makes sense to provide these essential nutrients alongside 5-HTP to enhance its conversion to serotonin.

St John's Wort

St John's Wort (*Hypericum perforatum*) is becoming the top natural treatment for mild to moderate depression, with all the benefits of prescription antidepressants, and none of the side-effects, at a tenth of the cost. Fifteen medical studies have now shown that it works, in some cases better than drugs. How it works is a bit of a mystery. One of its actions is to stop the body breaking down serotonin, the key brain chemical that controls mood. It also has a mild anti-anxiety effect; it has been shown to help sleep and can reduce PMS. For the maximum antidepressant effect, you need 300mg of a standardised extract containing 0.3 per cent hypericin (the active ingredient) 3 times a day. While some people report immediate improvement, it usually takes up to 3 weeks to notice a result.

While 5-HTP or St John's Wort are worth supplementing if you are prone to depression, a good memory- and mood-enhancing supplement may be helpful for general support.

Week 6

MEMORY AND MOOD **Action Plan**

DOs

- Eat a serving of fish at least every other day – particularly oily 'fish with teeth' such as sardines, salmon, herring, tuna, mackerel.

- Use cold-pressed sunflower, pumpkin or flax oil on salads – a blend of oils is best.

- Eat 1 heaped tablespoon of ground seeds daily – on cereal, soups, salads or casseroles.

- Eat plenty of B vitamin-rich foods – wholegrains, beans, lentils, fish, seeds and vegetables.

- Eat plenty of zinc-rich foods – nuts, seeds and wholegrains.

And as always . . .

1 heaped tablespoon of ground seeds or 1 tablespoon of cold-pressed seed oil.

2 servings of beans, lentils, quinoa, tofu (soya), or 'seed' vegetables.

3 pieces of fresh fruit such as apples, pears, bananas, berries, melon or citrus fruit.

4 servings of wholegrains such as rice, millet, rye, oats, corn or quinoa.

5 servings of dark green, leafy and root vegetables such as watercress, carrots, sweet potatoes, broccoli, spinach, green beans, peas and peppers.

6 glasses of water, diluted juices, herb or fruit teas.

7 Eat whole, organic, raw food as much as you can.

8 Avoid any form of sugar, white, refined or processed food with chemical additives.

9 Avoid all stimulants – coffee, tea, cigarettes.

10 Relax during your meal and chew your food well.

Week 6

DON'Ts

■ Avoid alcohol – limit your intake to no more than 2 units, 3 times this week.

■ Avoid all fried food.

■ Avoid processed fats such as margarine and any foods containing them.

MEMORY AND MOOD Menus

Below are some meal recommendations for Week 6. You can of course use or adapt recipes from other weeks which comply to the current 'Dos and Don'ts'.

Breakfast
● Choose from:
● Ultimate Power Breakfast (page 174)
● Get Up & Go (page 213) blended with skimmed or soya milk and a banana
● Breakfast Omelettes (page 178)
● Mixed Cereal Muesli with Grated Apples or Pears (page 176)

Other recipes can be taken from *The Optimum Nutrition Cookbook* (Piatkus, 1999), which I co-authored with Judy Ridgway.

Lunch
● Choose from:
● Hot Sour Prawn Soup (page 186)
● Stuffed Sardines Italian-style (page 192)
● Tomato Salad with Green Lentils and Sesame Tofu Dressing (page 190)

Other recommended recipes, taken from *The Optimum Nutrition Cookbook*, include: Carrot Soup in the Raw; Jacket Potato with Tofu Topping; Danish Herrings on Rye with Gherkins and Beetroot; Rainbow Vegetables with Avocado Dressing.

Dinner
Choose from:
● Thai Baked Fish with Steam-fried Vegetables (page 203)
● Red Mullet Baked in a Paper Case (page 207)
● Chickpea Crumble with Leafy Avocado Salad (page 208)

Week 6

Other recommended recipes, taken from *The Optimum Nutrition Cookbook*, include: Teriyaki Salmon with Tossed Steam-fry Vegetable Noodles; Potato, Coriander and Courgette Pie; Sesame Grilled Chicken on Celeriac Mash with Green Beans; Oriental Seafood with Sushi Rice.

MEMORY AND MOOD **Supplements**

As always	BREAKFAST	LUNCH	DINNER
Multi-vitamin/mineral	2		
Vitamin C 1,000mg	2		
Antioxidant complex	2		

Add			
'Smart nutrient' formula	2		

Optional

- Take 400mg × 2 of EPA/DHA if you scored above 6 in the Essential Fat questionnaire on page 146.

Optional to continue	BREAKFAST	LUNCH	DINNER
Chromium 200mcg	1		
Digestive enzymes	1	1	1
Herbal Aloe Detox	1 tablespoon	1 tablespoon	
Essential Balance	1 tablespoon		

MEMORY AND MOOD **Awareness Exercise**

What good food is to the body, meditation is to the mind. Studies on meditation have shown that the positive effects are greater than those gained simply from sleep. These include increased peace and contentment, better responsiveness to stressful events and quicker recovery, reduced heart rate and blood pressure, slowed rate of breathing and more stable brainwave patterns. Meditation has also been shown to prevent the depression of the body's immune responses that occur with stress. People who practise meditation on a regular basis have been found to be less anxious, and there is little doubt that meditation and relaxation techniques are effective in dealing with anxiety, stress and insomnia.

However, the true power of meditation in generating energy, clarity and peace goes beyond these beneficial effects measured in clinical studies. No one would doubt that stress is a mental as well as a physical phenomenon. The true power of meditation is its effects on gaining control over the mind.

Focusing the Mind

The starting point for meditation involves focusing your thoughts on one object, be it a sound, a candle flame or the breath. With this one pointed concentration the power of the mind seems to grow, and with that, your mental energy intensifies. This is the opposite to the experience of being stressed and exhausted, in which the nature of the mind is to flit from one thing to another leaving a trail of panic.

During this week set aside 10 minutes every day to practise meditation.

- **Sit in a quiet place and adopt a comfortable posture** with your spine straight. If you are sitting cross-legged on the floor you may find it helpful to straighten your spine by tucking a firm cushion under your pelvis.

- **Let go of any tension** in your body and feel your spine elongate.

- **Become aware of your breath** and start Dia-Kath breathing (see page 59) for 9 breaths.

- **Now let your breathing find its own rhythm.** Visualise your breath as a circle. As you inhale, move your awareness to the top of the circle. Become aware of a brief pause at the top of the circle as your breath pauses. As you exhale, move your awareness to the bottom of the circle. Become aware of a brief pause at the bottom of the circle, before the next inhalation. Bring your awareness to the place from where your breath arises. With each exhalation, bring your awareness to the place to where your breath goes.

- **Whenever your mind wanders, bring it back to the breath.** There is no need to resist your thoughts as such – simply become aware that your focus has shifted to your thoughts and bring it back to the breath.

- **Every day practise meditation** for 10 minutes ideally on rising or at the end of the day.

Week 6

- **Whenever you are stressed**, in an unpleasant mood or mentally exhausted, practise meditation by sitting quietly for 5 or more minutes.

If you'd like to deepen your experience of meditation, see page 214 for details of meditation courses.

WEEK 6 Psychocalisthenics Exercises

Cobra

These 3 exercises complete the full routine which you can now use every day as part of your superhealthy lifestyle.

Breathing *Inhale*, up, 6 counts: *Hold breath*, 3 counts: *Exhale*, down, 6 counts: *Hold*, 3 counts

Repeat ×3

Points to note Begin the Cobra by using the long muscles of the back to raise your upper body, then let your arms support you. Keep your pelvis on the floor, letting your arms bend at the elbows. Drop your shoulders and stretch your elbows down a little toward the floor and back toward your hip bones. This pulls your shoulders down even further and stretches the muscles at the sides of the neck. Relax the buttocks and look straight ahead.

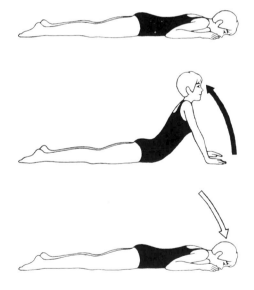

Week 6

Pendulum

Sit back on your heels, enjoy the stretch of your back, and stand up

Foot position Feet together

Breathing *Inhale*, swing left leg forward, 1 count: *Exhale*, swing left leg back, 1 count: *Rest*, 2 counts: *Inhale*, swing right leg forward, 1 count: *Exhale*, swing right leg back, 1 count

Repeat ×9 for each leg

Points to note The leg taking your weight is unlocked at the knee, the foot spread and relaxed on the floor. Your awareness is in your *Kath* or balance point. Focus your sight on something directly ahead of you. Sense the weight and relaxation of the swinging leg and let your arms naturally follow, relaxed and loose.

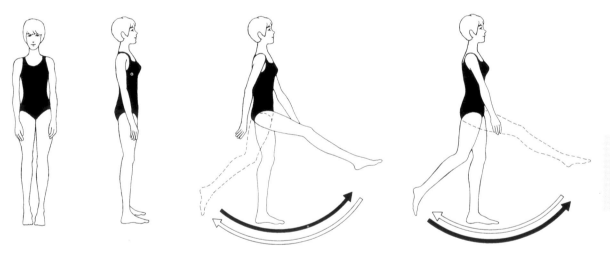

Completo

Foot position 2 foot-widths

Breathing *Inhale*, step in to 1½ foot-widths, 3 counts: *Exhale*, drop and bounce 3 times, 3 counts: *Hold breath*, step back (left, then right) and raise hips, 3 counts: *Inhale*, dive and scoop, 3 counts: *Inhale*, raise and drop hips, 3 counts: *Inhale*, raise and drop hips, 3 counts: *Hold breath*, jump forward, 1 count: *Exhale*, stand up, 2 counts

Repeat ×1

Points to note Drop down into a crouched position at the beginning of Completo, with your palms flat on the floor. This will steady your body during the bounces as you pump all the air out of your lungs. Your hands are ready to take your weight as you step back. Stepping back first left (count 1), then right (count 2), keep your hips low. Then on count 3, lift your hips as high as possible in preparation for the dive and scoop. Look back at your toes when your pelvis is raised, and look straight ahead when your pelvis is down. Your entire body from head to toe will be flexed. When your pelvis is up, feel for the maximum stretch in the backs of your legs by simultaneously reaching up with your tail bone and down with your heels. Keep the sequence of movements fluid and smooth.

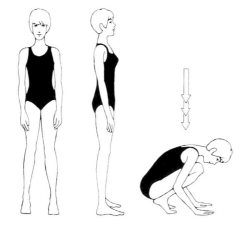

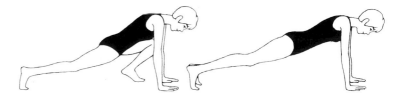

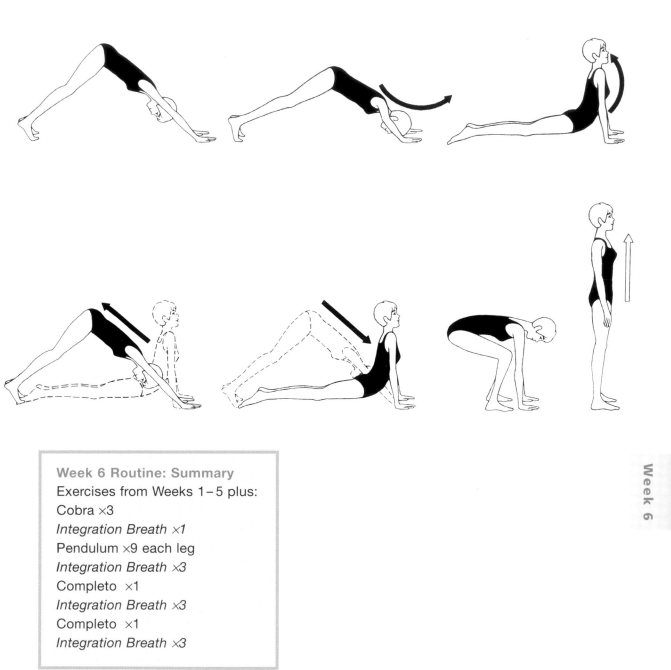

Week 6

Week 6 Routine: Summary
Exercises from Weeks 1–5 plus:
Cobra ×3
Integration Breath ×1
Pendulum ×9 each leg
Integration Breath ×3
Completo ×1
Integration Breath ×3
Completo ×1
Integration Breath ×3

You now have the instructions for the complete *Psychocalisthenics* exercise routine as summarised on pages 30–1.

Congratulations! You may be healthier now than you've ever been before. Using the exercises and recipes that you've learned in this book you'll find it easy to maintain your new superhealth. You can always repeat one or more of the weeks if there is an area you need to pay particular attention to. Part 4 will show you just how easy it is to stay in great shape and maximise your health.

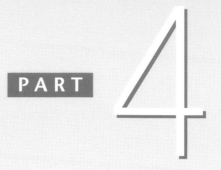

STAYING SUPERHEALTHY

Reassess Your Health

One-to-one Support

Superhealth for Life

Reassess Your Health

Now you've completed your 6 Weeks to Superhealth programme, how healthy are you? Check yourself on the Superhealth Questionnaire below, then compare your scores to those of your original questionnaire on page 14.

Score the questionnaire as follows:

0 for rarely or never

1 for sometimes

2 for frequently or always

Mark down your total for each of the 6 sections and your overall score.

1. Energy Check

- Are you still sleepy 20 minutes after getting up?
- Do you need tea, coffee, a cigarette or something to get you going in the morning?
- Do you crave sweet foods, bread, cereal, popcorn or pasta?
- Do you feel like you 'need' an alcoholic drink on most days?
- Are you overweight and unable to shift the extra pounds?
- Do you often have energy slumps during the day or after meals?
- Do you often have mood swings or difficulty concentrating?
- Do you get dizzy or irritable if you go 6 hours without food?
- Do you often find you over-react to stress?
- Is your energy now less than it used to be?

Section Total

2. Digestion Check

- Do you fail to chew your food thoroughly?
- Do you suffer from bad breath?
- Do you get a burning sensation in your stomach or regularly use indigestion tablets?
- Do you have a feeling of fullness in your stomach?
- Do you find it difficult digesting fatty foods?

- Do you get diarrhoea? ☐
- Do you get constipation? ☐
- Do you often get a bloated stomach or feel nauseous? ☐
- Do you often belch or pass wind? ☐
- Do you fail to have a bowel movement at least once a day? ☐

Section Total ☐

3. Hormone Check

Women

- Do you use the contraceptive pill? ☐
- Do you often suffer from cyclical mood swings or depression? ☐
- Do you experience cyclical water retention? ☐
- Do you especially crave foods premenstrually? ☐
- Have you at any time been bothered with problems affecting your reproductive organs (ovaries, womb)? ☐
- Do you have fertility problems, difficulty conceiving or a history of miscarriage? ☐
- Do you suffer from breast tenderness? ☐
- Do you experience cramps or other menstrual irregularities? ☐
- Are your periods often irregular or heavy? ☐
- Do you suffer from reduced libido or loss of interest in sex? ☐

Section Total ☐

Men

- Have you had a vasectomy? ☐
- Are you gaining weight? ☐
- Do you often suffer from mood swings or depression? ☐
- Have you at any time been bothered with problems affecting your reproductive organs (prostate or testes)? ☐
- Do you suffer from reduced libido or loss of interest in sex? ☐
- Do you suffer from impotence? ☐

- Do you awake less frequently with a morning erection or have difficulty maintaining an erection? ☐
- Do you suffer from fatigue or loss of energy? ☐
- Have you had a drop in your motivation and drive? ☐
- Do you feel that you are ageing prematurely? ☐

Section Total ☐

4. Detoxification Check

- Do you suffer from headaches or migraine? ☐
- Do you have watery or itchy eyes or swollen, red or sticky eyelids or bags or dark circles under your eyes? ☐
- Do you have itchy ears, earache, ear infections, drainage from the ears or ringing in the ears? ☐
- Do you suffer from excessive mucus, a stuffy nose or sinus problems? ☐
- Do you suffer from acne or skin rashes or hives? ☐
- Do you sweat a lot and have a strong body odour? ☐
- Do you have joint or muscle aches or pains? ☐
- Do you have a sluggish metabolism and find it hard to lose weight, or are you underweight and find it hard to gain weight? ☐
- Do you suffer from nausea or vomiting? ☐
- Do you have a bitter taste in your mouth or a furry tongue? ☐

Section Total ☐

5. Immunity Check

- Do you get more than 3 colds a year? ☐
- Do you get a stomach bug each year? ☐
- Do you find it hard to shift an infection (cold or otherwise)? ☐
- Are you prone to thrush or cystitis? ☐
- Do you take at least one course of antibiotics each year? ☐
- Is there any history of cancer in your family? ☐
- Do the glands in your neck, armpits or groin feel tender? ☐

- Do you suffer from allergy problems? ☐
- Do you take any drugs or medicines? ☐
- Do you have an inflammatory disease such as eczema, asthma or arthritis? ☐

Section Total ☐

6. Memory and Mood Check

- Is your memory deteriorating? ☐
- Do you find it hard to concentrate and often get confused? ☐
- Are you depressed? ☐
- Do you become anxious easily or wake up with a feeling of anxiety? ☐
- Does stress leave you feeling exhausted? ☐
- Do you have mood swings and easily become angry or irritable? ☐
- Are you lacking in motivation? ☐
- Do you feel like you're 'out of control' of things? ☐
- Do you have misperceptions where things don't look or sound right or you feel distant or disconnected? ☐
- Do you suffer from insomnia? ☐

Section Total ☐

Overall Total ☐

	Before	After
Energy Check	☐	☐
Digestion Check	☐	☐
Hormone Check	☐	☐
Detoxification Check	☐	☐
Immunity Check	☐	☐
Memory and Mood Check	☐	☐
Total Score	☐	☐

Percentage Improvement (Before/After $\times$ 100) = ☐

5. **Meditation/contemplation** – Make sure you leave some time each day to meditate or contemplate, perhaps by listening to a favourite piece of music or going for a walk in the park.

6. **Diet** – Follow the basic guidelines for the Superhealth Diet (see page 20) with particular emphasis on the following areas. In addition, stay away from foods you are allergic to.

7. **Sugar** – Stay away from sugar and foods which contain it. Sweeten foods with fresh or dried fruit and dilute fruit juices with water.

8. **Fat** – Cut right back on meat and dairy products, substituting vegetarian foods and fish. Avoid foods that contain hydrogenated fats and eat a tablespoon of ground seeds or seed oil every day to ensure an optimal intake of essential fats.

9. **Fruit and vegetables** – Eat loads. Have a piece of fruit in the morning, take fruit to work for snacks and keep fruit at home for when you are feeling peckish. Fill yourself up with vegetables.

10. **Supplements** – Take them every day. A good supplement programme may contain the following:

Multi-vitamin/mineral	2 a day
Vitamin C 1,000mg and bioflavonoids	2 a day
Antioxidant formula	2 a day
'Smart' nutrients	2 a day

6 Weeks to Superhealth Revisited

The 6 Weeks to Superhealth strategy is a wonderful way to give your health a quantum leap. Consider doing it every year as part of your new year's resolution. If a particular week was important for you, perhaps because you had a high score in that area or it challenged you in particular areas of addiction, consider repeating the recommendations for that week.

You can also see Recommended Reading on page 218 to give you further knowledge and motivation.

PART 5

RECIPES, SHOPPING AND RESOURCES

Superhealth Recipes

BREAKFASTS

ultimate power breakfast

Not only does this recipe offer optimum nutrition, it's also a great way to meet your daily five-fruit requirement.

Instead of leaving fruit to go mouldy or mushy in a fruit bowl, the Ultimate Power Breakfast ensures that you get a head start at the beginning of the day. Any additional fruit eaten later on becomes an added bonus!

Here's how to put the Ultimate Power Breakfast together.

1 Blend 250g (9oz) low-fat, organic yoghurt with a variety of fruit in a food processor. Choose four or five fruits from the following:

bananas (we usually include two for carbohydrate content and to make the mixture thick and velvety)

kiwis

mangoes

berries (frozen in winter)

pears

apricots, peaches, nectarines, plums

figs

apple sauce (especially in winter when the choice of fruit diminishes)

dried fruit, soaked and reconstituted overnight (also a good winter choice)

2 Separately, finely grind 4–6 level tablespoons five-seed mix in an electric coffee grinder: the ideal mix is ½ tablespoon flax, and ½ teaspoon each of sesame, pumpkin, sunflower and hemp per tablespoon. Mix these whole seeds ahead of time and store in the fridge.

3 Stir the ground seeds into the yoghurt and fruit mix. Then add 2–3 tablespoons cold-pressed mixed seed oil.

4 Blend in a food processor until the mixture has a smooth, creamy texture. Add water or milk if you want to drink it. Otherwise serve in a soup bowl. Enjoy immediately to avoid discoloration and oxidation.

> • All superhealth recipes serve 2

berry booster

This makes a wonderful start to the day in summer when there are plenty of berries available. Serve on its own or add to your usual muesli or porridge. Choose individual berries or mix and match to get the best flavours.

250g (9oz) low-fat natural live yoghurt
225g (8oz) berries (e.g. strawberries, blueberries, raspberries, blackcurrants or blackberries)
2 tablespoons wheatgerm
2 level tablespoons five-seed mix (see previous page), freshly ground

1 Place all the ingredients in a blender and process until smooth. Serve at once.

Anton Mosimann's oat muesli with fruit

Muesli was invented in Switzerland so it is not surprising that this world-renowned Swiss chef should have come up with the king of muesli recipes. Here it is:

2 tablespoons rolled oats
1 dessertspoon oat germ and bran
50ml (2fl oz) warmed skimmed milk
75g (3oz) low-fat natural live yoghurt
2 tablespoons honey
1 tablespoon lemon juice
½ red apple, washed and grated with the skin on
½ green apple, washed and grated with the skin on
2 tablespoons toasted hazelnuts, chopped
150g (5½oz) berries (e.g. strawberries, raspberries, currants and blueberries)
sprigs of mint, to garnish

1 Soak the rolled oats, oatgerm and bran in the warm milk for at least 2 hours.
2 Stir in the yoghurt, honey and lemon juice. Next, add the freshly grated apples and chopped nuts, and fold into the mixture. Finally, add the berries and decorate with sprigs of mint.

mixed cereal muesli with grated apples or pears

You can add variety by using the different kinds of flaked cereals on sale in specialist health-food and organic shops to make muesli with different tastes and textures. Avoid wheat or rye flakes if you have a problem with gluten.

75–100g (3–3½oz) mixed cereal flakes (e.g. wheat, rye, oats, millet, rice)

1 tablespoon raisins

2 level tablespoons five-seed mix (see page 174), freshly ground

2 apples or pears, grated or finely chopped

a little lemon juice

150g (5½oz) low-fat natural live yoghurt

1 Place the mixed cereal flakes in two soup bowls, add the raisins and 100–125ml (3½–4fl oz) water. Soak the flakes overnight.

2 Sprinkle on the ground seed mix. Grate or chop the fruit and mix with a little lemon juice to prevent discoloration.

3 Spoon the fruit on to the muesli, top with yoghurt and serve at once.

oat porridge

Rolled or porridge oats make the quickest porridge. This is usually ready in 3–5 minutes, depending on the size of the flakes. You can also use oatmeal but it takes longer to cook.

250–275ml (9–9½fl oz) skimmed milk, soya or rice milk

250–275ml (9–9½fl oz) water

75g (3oz) porridge oats

2 teaspoons honey

1 tablespoon mixed flax (linseed) and pumpkin seeds, freshly ground

1 Pour the milk and the water into a saucepan and sprinkle in the oats. Bring to the boil and simmer for 4–5 minutes, stirring all the time.

2 Serve with the honey and the ground seed mixture.

millet or rice flake porridge

Both these flaked cereals cook as quickly, if not faster, than porridge oats. The resulting porridges tend to be smoother (more like semolina) and without such a definite flavour, so flavourings are important.

75g (3oz) flaked rice or millet
400–450ml (14–16fl oz) half-and-half skimmed or soya milk and water
nutmeg or vanilla essence (to taste)
2 teaspoons honey
1 tablespoon five-seed mix (see page 174), freshly ground

1 Cook in just the same way as the Oat Porridge, adding the nutmeg or vanilla flavouring at the beginning of the cooking time.

simple fruit muesli

If you keep using different fruits you'll never get bored with muesli.

75–100g (3–3½oz) oat flakes or porridge oats
2 dessertspoons wheatgerm
250g (9oz) fruit (e.g. sliced bananas, chopped mangoes or pawpaw, or soft fruit)
150g (5½oz) low-fat natural live yoghurt
1 heaped tablespoon five-seed mix (see page 174), freshly ground, or mixed chopped almonds and hazelnuts

1 Place the oat flakes or porridge oats in two soup bowls and cover with 100–125ml (3½–4fl oz) water. Leave to soak overnight.
2 Add the wheatgerm and top with the fruit and yoghurt.
3 Sprinkle on the ground seeds or chopped nuts, and serve at once.

healthy scrambled eggs

While eggs are rather high in fat, they are also a good source of protein and can add variety to your diet. Serve them occasionally as part of a more substantial breakfast.

2 large free-range eggs
2 tablespoons skimmed or soya milk
2 tablespoons freshly chopped parsley
a knob of butter
2 slices whole rye toast

1 Beat the eggs with the milk and parsley.
2 Melt the butter in a small saucepan. Pour in the egg mixture and cook slowly over a low heat, stirring constantly. Serve on whole rye toast.

breakfast omelettes

This omelette is a very quick way of serving eggs. Fillings add extra nutrients, as well as interest.

3 free-range eggs
3 tablespoons skimmed or soya milk
a knob of butter
a filling (e.g. 2 tablespoons mixed beansprouts, 1 finely chopped tomato, ½ finely chopped red pepper, 2 tablespoons canned sweetcorn or Mexicorn)

1 Beat the eggs and milk in a bowl. Heat the butter in a small non-stick frying pan and pour in the egg mixture. Carefully stir the egg to fold the mixture a little.
2 When it is nearly set, sprinkle on your chosen filling and fold over. Cut in half to serve.

LUNCHES

winter salad platter with tangy cucumber dressing

Most root vegetables are delicious if they are simply grated and eaten raw. This way you also receive their full vitamin content. For a change, try celeriac, turnip, kholrabi or white radish in place of one of the vegetables used here.

The lightly toasted nuts and seeds add flavour and a crunchy texture but take care not to burn them.

TANGY CUCUMBER DRESSING

7–10cm (3–4in) length of cucumber, chopped

25g (1oz) low-fat natural live yoghurt

2 spring onions, roughly chopped

½ clove garlic, peeled and chopped

2 teaspoons cider vinegar

½ teaspoon Dijon mustard

a few drops Worcester sauce

2 teaspoons freshly chopped dill

½ teaspoon celery seeds (optional)

WINTER SALAD PLATTER

2 heads chicory, trimmed and sliced

100g (3½oz) cabbage greens or sprout tops, very finely shredded

200g (7oz) carrots, peeled and finely grated

1 teaspoon lemon juice

2 medium-sized uncooked beetroot, peeled and finely grated

200g (7oz) uncooked parsnip, peeled and finely grated

2 tablespoons mixed lightly toasted sunflower seeds and flaked almonds or pine nuts

1 Start by making the Tangy Cucumber Dressing. Place all the ingredients in a blender and process until smooth. If possible, refrigerate for an hour or so (in order to blend the flavours). Whisk lightly with a fork before using.

2 Mix the sliced chicory and cabbage greens together and arrange on two serving plates.

3 Mix the carrot with a little lemon juice to prevent it from discoloring.

4 Arrange small mounds of the carrot and grated vegetables on top of the cabbage greens and chicory. Then pour on the Tangy Cucumber Dressing, sprinkle with the toasted seeds and nuts and serve at once.

Brussels sprouts and nut salad

This wonderfully crunchy, detoxifying salad makes a good light lunch. Follow it with fresh fruit or dates stuffed with low-fat soft cheese.

150g (5½oz) Brussels sprouts, trimmed and thinly sliced
12 radishes, trimmed and sliced
3cm (1½ in) length of cucumber, diced
50g (2oz) lightly toasted almonds or cashews
2 tablespoons freshly chopped parsley
2 tablespoons cold-pressed mixed seed oil
2 tablespoons lemon juice

1 Prepare the vegetables and mix together in a bowl. Divide the mixture between two serving bowls and top with the toasted nuts and parsley.
2 Mix the seed oil and lemon juice together, pour over the top of the salad mix and serve.

red cabbage and mixed vegetable salad with tofu

You can make this colourful, crunchy salad at any time of the year. Serve it with rye bread.

75g (3oz) red cabbage, chopped
75g (3oz) broccoli florets, chopped
2 medium carrots, scrubbed and grated
2 sticks celery, sliced
2 spring onions, chopped
150g (5½oz) smoked or marinated tofu, diced

DRESSING
2 tablespoons cold-pressed mixed seed oil
1 tablespoon lemon juice or cider vinegar
freshly ground black pepper (to taste)

1 Combine all the salad ingredients in a large bowl.
2 Mix the dressing ingredients together and pour over the top of the salad separately. Toss together and serve at once.

chicken salad with horseradish sauce

The horseradish sauce in this filling, main-course salad recipe is both piquant and refreshing. It would also make a good dressing for much simpler side salads, to serve with roasts or grills.

2 Little Gem lettuces, shredded

200–250g (7–9oz) cooked chicken meat without the skin, cut into chunks

2 medium potatoes, steamed in their skins, peeled, cooled and sliced

1 eating apple, cubed

5cm (2in) length of cucumber, sliced

8 cherry tomatoes, halved

a few sprigs of fresh parsley or dill

paprika pepper (to taste)

HORSERADISH SAUCE

3 heaped tablespoons low-fat natural live yoghurt

1 tablespoon horseradish sauce

3 tablespoons lemon juice

3 tablespoons skimmed milk or water

1 Place the shredded lettuce on two serving plates. Arrange the chicken, sliced potatoes, apple, cucumber and tomatoes on top of the lettuce.

2 Mix all the Horseradish Sauce ingredients in a cup and spoon over the salads. Decorate with the fresh herbs and a sprinkling of paprika pepper.

steam-fried vegetables with green curry paste

Don't worry if you don't have all the ingredients listed for this very versatile dish – simply substitute the vegetables that you do have to hand. Cauliflower, beans, broccoli, sugar snap peas, mangetout and asparagus can all be used.

We have used a proprietary Thai green curry paste for this recipe. You can, of course, make up your own Thai mix of spices but it is quite expensive to buy all the ingredients and, unless you regularly make Thai dishes, they can go to waste. Look out for brands which do not use any additives – check the ingredients list.

1 onion, peeled and sliced

2 cloves garlic, peeled and chopped

1 teaspoon extra-virgin olive oil

2–3 tablespoons water or vegetable stock

2–3 tablespoons green curry paste (to taste)

1 red pepper, seeded and cut into strips

6–8 baby courgettes, cut in half lengthways, or 1 large courgette, cut into sticks

6–8 patty pan courgettes, trimmed and cut in half

300g (10½oz) tofu, cubed

1 carrot, shaved with a large potato peeler

100g (3½oz) brown cap or shiitake mushrooms, sliced

2 tablespoons coconut milk

150g (5½oz) beansprouts

fresh coriander (to garnish)

1 Quickly steam-fry the onion and garlic in the oil and then in the water or stock for 2–3 minutes. Stir in the green curry paste and add the pepper, courgettes and patty pan courgettes. Continue to steam-fry for another 3–4 minutes.

2 Add all the remaining ingredients, except the beansprouts and coriander, and toss carefully in the pan juices. Cook until the vegetables are cooked but still firm to the bite.

3 Stir in the beansprouts, toss and serve with rice or noodles. Garnish with sprigs of fresh coriander.

lemon chicken on leafy asparagus salad

If you like, you can use firm fish fillets such as tuna or salmon or fried tofu, in place of the chicken in this lovely warm recipe. Serve with good crusty rolls.

1 large chicken breast, skinned and boned

juice of ½ lemon

1 clove garlic, peeled and crushed

1 stick lemongrass or 1 teaspoon dried chopped lemongrass

freshly ground black pepper (to taste)

1 teaspoon cold-pressed mixed seed oil

100g (3½oz) asparagus spears

8 baby courgettes

100g (3½oz) mixed salad leaves

1 tablespoon lightly toasted flaked almonds or pine nuts

1 Cut the chicken into thin strips, put it into a non-metallic bowl and mix it with the lemon juice, garlic, lemongrass, black pepper and cold-pressed mixed seed oil. Cover and refrigerate until required.

2 Place the asparagus and courgettes in the top of a steamer over boiling water and cook for about 5 minutes to soften slightly.

3 Arrange the mixed leaves on two serving plates and top with the lightly cooked vegetables.

4 Brush a non-stick wok with a little more oil and steam-fry the chicken pieces, using the strained marinade to moisten the pan after a minute or two.

5 Cover with a lid and leave on the heat for about 8 minutes until the chicken is cooked through.

6 Spoon the chicken and the pan juices over the salad. Sprinkle with the nuts and serve at once.

Provençal tuna salad in a bun

Known as Pain Bagnat *in the South of France, these buns are more of a meal than a snack!*

2 large sesame buns, split in half
1–2 tablespoons extra-virgin olive oil
8–10 soft lettuce leaves
1 good-sized Continental tomato or 2 ordinary tomatoes, sliced
1 × 100g (3½oz) can of tuna in olive oil, drained and flaked
1 very small onion, peeled and thinly sliced
½ small red pepper, seeded and cut into rings
12 black olives (optional)

1 Brush each half of the bun with olive oil. Place the bases on a board and arrange the lettuce leaves and tomato slices on them. Next, add the tuna, onion and pepper rings.
2 Add more olive oil to taste and dot with black olives, if using. Place the second half of the bun on top and press down well. Serve at once. Warn everyone about the olive stones!

sweet potato and carrot soup

This wonderfully creamy soup couldn't be easier to make. Its bright orange colour reflects the high level of carotenoids in these year-round vegetables. A good alternative to sweet potato is butternut squash.

250g (9oz) sweet potatoes, peeled and finely chopped
250g (9oz) carrots, scrubbed and finely chopped
100ml (3½fl oz) canned coconut milk
½–1 clove garlic (to taste), crushed
black pepper (to taste)

1 Boil the sweet potatoes and carrots in 350ml (12fl oz) water for about 15 minutes until soft.
2 Purée the soup in a blender with the coconut milk, garlic and black pepper, then serve.

gazpacho

Choose the ripest and most flavoursome tomatoes you can find for this famous Andalucian soup.
If you are not sure of the quality of your tomatoes, add some good tomato purée.

225g (8oz) ripe tomatoes, roughly chopped
1 large clove of garlic, peeled and chopped
4–5 spring onions, trimmed and chopped
½ red pepper, seeded and chopped
5cm (2in) length cucumber, roughly chopped
225ml (8fl oz) passata
juice of 1 lemon
1½ tablespoons extra-virgin olive oil
salt and freshly ground black pepper (to taste)

GARNISH
2.5cm (1in) cucumber, diced
¼ red or green pepper, seeded and diced
1 tablespoon freshly chopped spring onions

1 Place the tomatoes in a blender with the garlic and process for a minute. Add the rest of the vegetables and process again. Take care not to over-process – the soup should have quite a rough texture.
2 Transfer to a bowl and stir in the rest of the soup ingredients. Leave to stand in the fridge for 15–20 minutes. Prepare the cucumber, pepper and spring onion for the Garnish and serve sprinkled over the soup.

hot sour prawn soup

Tamarind paste gives this South-East Asian soup a deep lemony flavour. You can buy tamarind in ethnic grocers and some specialist delicatessens. If you cannot find it, try lemon juice.

600ml (1 pint) chicken stock
½ teaspoon tamarind paste
1 small fresh green chilli
1 dried red chilli
1 piece lemongrass
2 slices fresh lime
2 small carrots, peeled and sliced diagonally
75g (3oz) broccoli, broken into small florets
50g (2oz) pak choy or Chinese greens, coarsely sliced
4–6 spring onions, sliced diagonally
1 tablespoon soy sauce
4–6 large King prawns, cooked and peeled
plenty of fresh coriander leaves

1 Pour the stock into a saucepan and add the tamarind paste, chillies, lemongrass and lime. Bring to the boil and simmer for about 10–15 minutes.

2 Prepare the vegetables, add the carrots and broccoli to the pan and continue to simmer for a further 2–3 minutes.

3 Now add all the remaining ingredients except the coriander. Return to the boil and serve garnished with plenty of fresh coriander leaves.

spicy lentil and watercress soup

By adding the watercress to the soup at the very last minute you will get every bit of benefit from its nutrients. Put it all in — even the long stalks.

50g (2oz) red split lentils, picked over and washed

1 small onion, peeled and chopped

1 small carrot, peeled and chopped

600ml (1 pint) vegetable stock or water

1 bay leaf

½ teaspoon mild curry powder

¼ teaspoon dried thyme

¼ teaspoon celery salt

freshly ground black pepper (to taste)

50g (2oz) watercress

1 Place all the ingredients except the watercress in a saucepan and bring to the boil. Cover with a lid, reduce the heat and simmer for 30 minutes.

2 Remove the bay leaf and purée in a blender. Add the watercress, whizz quickly and reheat. Serve at once.

chunky bean and kale soup

This main course soup is excellent poured over a hunk of day-old bread in the Tuscan manner. Alternatively, you can serve it over toasted polenta squares or with rye bread.

1 teaspoon extra-virgin olive oil
1 medium onion, peeled and chopped
2 sticks celery, sliced
1 carrot, peeled and diced
500ml (16fl oz) well-flavoured vegetable stock
150g (5½oz) cooked or canned red kidney beans
150g (5½oz) curly kale, shredded
1 tablespoon tomato purée
½ teaspoon dried oregano
1 clove garlic, peeled and finely chopped
salt and freshly ground black pepper (to taste)

1 Heat the oil in a large saucepan and add all the fresh vegetables except the kale. Stir over a very low heat for 2–3 minutes to release all the flavours.
2 Add the stock and bring to the boil. Reduce the heat and cook for 15 minutes.
3 Mash half the kidney beans with a potato masher and add to the soup with the whole beans, the shredded kale, tomato purée, herbs and seasonings and continue cooking for another 10 minutes. Very tough kale may need a little longer to soften.

rocket salad with chickpeas in tahini dressing

You can use any bitter leaves for this spicy salad. Try it with the cultivated dandelion leaves you can often buy at Greek delis or with watercress or even mustard and cress.

a handful of rocket, approximately 25g (1oz)
3–4 large sprigs broadleaf parsley
100g (3½oz) canned chickpeas, drained weight
½ red pepper, seeded and very finely chopped

TAHINI DRESSING
1 heaped teaspoon tahini paste
2 teaspoons cold-pressed mixed seed oil
1 teaspoon lemon juice

1 Arrange the rocket and parsley on two small plates or shallow entrée dishes and sprinkle with the chickpeas and chopped red pepper.

2 Mix all the Tahini Dressing ingredients together in a cup with 2 teaspoons water and spoon a little over each salad. Serve at once.

Bulgarian salad with feta cheese

This simple but very effective starter appears on the menu at almost every Bulgarian restaurant, hence the title.

2 tomatoes

1 small cucumber

1 red or green pepper

4 spring onions, chopped

3 tablespoons freshly chopped mint

freshly ground black pepper (to taste)

juice of 1 lemon

75g (3oz) Feta cheese, crumbled

1 Cut the tomatoes, cucumber and pepper into very small dice and mix with the chopped spring onions and mint, retaining a few sprigs for decoration. Spoon the mixture into two bowls.

2 Sprinkle with black pepper and lemon juice. Top with the Feta cheese and serve decorated with the retained sprigs of mint.

tomato salad with green lentils and sesame tofu dressing

The best green lentils come either from Puy in the Auvergne or from Castelluccio di Norcia in Umbria. Both these products have DOP (or denomination of origin status), which means that the lentils must come from the designated areas, and both varieties are very small and sweet.

35g (1¼oz) whole green lentils
2 large Continental tomatoes, sliced

SESAME TOFU DRESSING
100g (3½oz) tofu
50ml (2fl oz) soya milk
1 clove garlic, crushed
1 tablespoon tahini
juice of ½ small lemon
½–1 teaspoon soy sauce (to taste)

1 Place the lentils in a saucepan and cover with 100ml (3½fl oz) water. Bring to the boil, cover and simmer over a low heat for 20–25 minutes until the lentils are almost cooked, but still *al dente*. Drain and leave to cool.

2 Place all the dressing ingredients in a blender and process quickly until the consistency is smooth and fairly runny.

3 Arrange the sliced tomatoes on individual plates and scatter the cooked lentils over the top. Spoon on the Sesame Tofu Dressing and serve.

smoked tofu on oriental glass noodles with shredded vegetables

This recipe makes an excellent starter, especially for a Thai meal. Shred the celeriac and carrot by cutting them first into thin slices, then into sticks.

600ml (1 pint) good vegetable stock
1 stick lemongrass, cut lengthways down the centre
1 clove of garlic, peeled and sliced
4 thin slices fresh root ginger, peeled
50g (2oz) carrots, peeled
50g (2oz) celeriac, peeled
50g (2oz) Chinese glass noodles or transparent vermicelli
50g (2oz) mangetout
4 spring onions, trimmed and sliced diagonally
3 teaspoons soy sauce
freshly ground black pepper (to taste)
150g/5oz smoked tofu, cut into strips
a few sprigs of fresh coriander

1 Put the stock in a large saucepan and add the lemongrass, garlic and ginger. Bring to the boil and simmer for about 10 minutes.

2 Prepare the carrots and celeriac and add to the pan. Continue to cook, uncovered, over a low to medium heat, for a further 3–4 minutes to soften the vegetables.

3 Place the glass noodles or vermicelli in a bowl and pour boiling water over them. Leave to stand for 3–4 minutes. Drain and add to the saucepan with the stock and vegetables. Add the mangetout, spring onions, soy sauce and seasoning and turn up the heat.

4 Boil for a couple of minutes to reduce the sauce a little and ladle into serving bowls. The mixture should be quite runny. Top with smoked tofu and garnish with a few sprigs of fresh coriander.

stuffed sardines Italian-style

Sardines are often overlooked but they, like mackerel and herring, are oily fish with good supplies of Omega 3. This dish from Sicily makes an excellent first course when you are entertaining, and a good lunch too. Ask your fishmonger to split the fish and remove the heads and backbones.

6 small or 4 larger sardines, approximately 400g (14oz), gutted

1 slice bread, approximately 1½oz, made into crumbs

40g (1½oz) Parmesan cheese, grated

1 tablespoon freshly chopped parsley

1 teaspoon freshly chopped basil

½ small beaten egg

a knob of butter

2 tablespoons lemon juice

a few sprigs of parsley (to garnish)

lemon wedges (to garnish)

1 Wash and prepare the fish if the fishmonger has not done so.

2 Mix the breadcrumbs, Parmesan cheese, parsley and basil with the beaten egg to make a firmish stuffing.

3 Lay the sardines flat, skin side down, and spread with the stuffing. Roll up each fish, starting from the neck end, and fix with half a cocktail stick.

4 Heat the butter in a small shallow pan and arrange the stuffed sardines in the pan. Fry gently for a minute or two, turning once.

5 Then add 4 tablespoons water and the lemon juice. Cover with a lid and cook for about 10 minutes, turning once again after 5 minutes.

6 Arrange the stuffed sardines on small serving plates and pour on the juices from the pan. Garnish with a few sprigs of parsley and lemon wedges.

DINNERS

salmon and monkfish kebabs with coriander and sunflower seed pesto

Here, the Pesto is more of a relish than a sauce. It is quite strong and it lifts this simple rice and fish dish into another dimension.

250g (9oz) piece monkfish
250g (9oz) salmon steak
juice of ½ lime
1 teaspoon extra-virgin olive oil
freshly ground black pepper (to taste)
100g (3½oz) rice or quinoa

CORIANDER AND SUNFLOWER SEED PESTO
a bunch of fresh coriander, approximately 25g (1oz)
25g (1oz) sunflower seeds
1 clove garlic, peeled
1 tablespoon cold-pressed mixed seed oil

1 Remove the skin and bones from the two fish and cut each one into six large chunks. Thread on to skewers. Mix the lime juice, oil and black pepper and pour evenly over the kebabs. Leave to stand until required for cooking.
2 Cook the rice or quinoa.
3 To make the Pesto, place the coriander, sunflower seeds and garlic in a food processor and process quickly. Do not allow the mixture to get too fine. Moisten with the cold-pressed seed oil and keep to one side.
4 Place the kebabs under a hot grill for 2½–3 minutes on each side until just cooked through. Do not allow the fish to overcook or it will be hard and unpleasant. Serve with the rice or quinoa and the Pesto.

roasted chicory and courgettes with salsa picante and bulgar

If you can find it, you can use Italian red radicchio in place of one of the heads of chicory to give more colour to this delicious roasted vegetable dish.

3 large heads of chicory
3 large or 5–6 small courgettes
a little extra-virgin olive oil
cooked bulgar

SALSA PICANTE
1 hard-boiled egg, finely chopped
2 tablespoons freshly chopped parsley
2 tablespoons freshly chopped chives
2 tablespoons capers, finely chopped
2 small green chillies, seeded and finely chopped
juice of ½ small lemon
2–3 tablespoons cold-pressed mixed seed oil

1 Cut each head of chicory into three pieces lengthways. Trim and slice the courgettes lengthways. Brush the vegetables with a little olive oil and place the chicory under a hot grill.

2 After 5 minutes, cover the tips of the chicory with a strip of foil to stop the leaves burning and add the courgette slices. Cook for another 8–10 minutes, turning the vegetables from time to time until lightly browned.

3 In the meantime, place all the Salsa ingredients in a bowl and mix well. When the vegetables are cooked, transfer to serving plates with the cooked bulgar. Spoon the Salsa over the top.

grilled carrot and tofu cakes with red peppers and fennel

You can use any kind of bread to make the breadcrumbs for this recipe.

2 large red peppers, seeded and cut into large pieces

200g (7oz) firm tofu, mashed with a potato masher

125g (4½oz) carrots, scrubbed and finely grated

50g (2oz) fresh rye or wholemeal breadcrumbs

25g (1oz) ground almonds

4–5 spring onions, trimmed and finely chopped

1 clove garlic, peeled and crushed

1 tablespoon soy sauce

freshly ground black pepper (to taste)

1 tablespoon sesame seeds

1 large head fennel, trimmed and thinly sliced

a few sprigs of fresh parsley

1 Prepare the peppers. Then take about a quarter of one pepper and chop very finely, keeping the other pieces on one side.

2 In a large bowl, mix the chopped pepper with the mashed tofu, grated carrots, breadcrumbs, ground almonds, spring onions and garlic. Stir in the soy sauce and black pepper. Then shape the mixture into four cakes and press down so that they are not too thick. Coat each side with a few sesame seeds.

3 Place the Carrot and Tofu Cakes on a piece of foil under a hot grill and add the pieces of red pepper and the sliced fennel. Cook for about 10 minutes on each side until the Carrot and Tofu Cakes are cooked and the vegetables are lightly browned.

4 Arrange the Carrot and Tofu Cakes on two serving plates with the grilled vegetables around them. Garnish with sprigs of fresh parsley.

flash-grilled tuna in lemon ginger marinade with quinoa and red pepper salsa

The best way to cook tuna is to flash-grill thin slices on a pre-heated ridged grill. This cooks the fish very fast and also leaves attractive markings across it.

300g (14oz) fresh tuna, cut into thin slices
cooked quinoa
a little cold-pressed mixed seed oil

MARINADE

juice and grated rind of 1 large or 1½ small lemons
50ml (2fl oz) dry white wine
2 tablespoons soy sauce
1 tablespoon saffron oil or ordinary olive oil with a pinch of saffron
6 spring onions, very finely chopped
1 clove garlic, peeled and crushed
1 tablespoon freshly grated ginger

RED PEPPER SALSA

1 red pepper, seeded and finely diced
½ small red chilli pepper, seeded and finely chopped
1 small cucumber, finely diced
2 tablespoons freshly chopped celery or fennel
3 tablespoons freshly chopped coriander
juice of ½ lemon
a little cold-pressed mixed seed oil (optional)

1 Place the tuna slices in a shallow non-metallic entrée dish. Mix all the Marinade ingredients together and pour over the fish. Leave to stand for at least an hour, turning from time to time.
2 Cook the quinoa and make the Red Pepper Salsa by simply mixing all the ingredients together in a bowl.
3 Remove the fish from the Marinade and pour the Marinade into a saucepan. Bring to the boil and leave to simmer while you cook the fish. Brush the tuna pieces with mixed seed oil and grill for 1½–2 minutes on each side.
4 Spoon the quinoa on to two serving plates and top with the tuna steaks. Serve with the cooked Marinade spooned over the top and the Salsa on the side.

grilled scallops with green sauce, julienne vegetables and rice noodles

This is another recipe where it pays to get all the preparation finished before you start cooking. Begin with the Green Sauce and then prepare the vegetables.

2 sticks celery, cut into lengths
100g (3½oz) carrots, peeled and sliced lengthways
100g (3½oz) small French beans, trimmed
1 small red pepper, seeded and sliced
6–8 spring onions, trimmed
50ml (2fl oz) well-flavoured vegetable stock
100–125g (3½–4½oz) rice noodles
12 scallops
a little extra-virgin olive oil

GREEN SAUCE

75g (3oz) spinach, washed and drained
a bunch of chives
25g (1oz) fresh coriander
15g (½oz) fresh basil
1 tablespoon fresh ginger, grated
250ml (9fl oz) well-flavoured vegetable stock
2 tablespoons Greek yoghurt
1–1½ tablespoons potato flour

1 To make the Green Sauce, place the spinach in a food processor with the herbs, ginger and stock and blend until smooth. Stir in the yoghurt and pour into a saucepan. Leave to one side until required.

2 Cut all the vegetables into long thin strips and steam–fry in a little stock for 1–2 minutes to soften slightly. Place on one side. Cook the rice noodles as indicated on the pack.

3 Brush the scallops with a little extra-virgin olive oil. Cook under a hot grill for 2½–3 minutes each side until they turn white. Take care not to overcook. If you are not sure, cut one scallop in half – it should be white all the way through.

4 As the scallops are cooking, place the Green Sauce over a medium heat and bring to the boil. Add the potato flour, stirring all the time, until the mixture boils and thickens.

5 Drain the noodles, toss with the steam-fried vegetables and spoon onto two serving plates. Arrange the cooked scallops on the noodles and drizzle the Green Sauce over the top. Alternatively, you could coat the plate with the sauce first.

spicy mackerel with couscous

North Africa provides the inspiration for this spicy sauce but take care with the harissa — some brands can be very hot indeed. Couscous is the traditional North African carbohydrate but you could use bulgar or quinoa instead.

a little extra-virgin olive oil
1 small onion, peeled and chopped
1 clove garlic, peeled and crushed
1 teaspoon ground cumin
½–1 teaspoon harissa or chilli powder
1 small red pepper, seeded and chopped
125g (4½oz) courgettes, diced
1 × 200g (7oz) can tomatoes
couscous
1 good-sized mackerel, approximately 300–350g (10½–12oz), cut into 2 fillets

1 Preheat the oven to 180°C/350°F/Gas 4.
2 Heat the oil in a small heavy-based saucepan and stir-fry the onion and garlic with the cumin and harissa or chilli powder for 1–2 minutes. Add the red pepper and courgettes and cook for another 2 minutes, stirring all the time.
3 Pour on the tomatoes and bring to the boil. Simmer for 10 minutes, stirring from time to time. Cook the couscous as directed on the packet.
4 Place the mackerel fillets on a non-stick baking tray and cover with foil. Bake in the oven for 10 minutes or until the fish is cooked through.
5 Arrange the fish on a mound of couscous and top with the sauce.

minted trout with grapefruit rice salad

It's important to use fresh mint for this recipe. Dried mint simply does not taste the same. Look for good, large fresh sprigs. The same goes for parsley, but it does not really matter whether you choose the curly English variety or the broadleaf Continental type.

2 trout, cleaned
a little extra-virgin olive oil
freshly ground black pepper (to taste)
3–4 sprigs fresh mint

GRAPEFRUIT RICE SALAD
100g (3½oz) long-grain rice
200–225ml (7–8fl oz) vegetable stock
1 large grapefruit, peeled
½ green pepper, seeded and very finely chopped
2 tablespoons freshly chopped parsley
1 tablespoon freshly chopped mint

1 Start by making the Grapefruit Rice Salad. Place the rice and stock in a saucepan and bring to the boil. Stir and cover. Reduce the heat and cook for 15–18 minutes until all the liquid has been absorbed and the rice is tender.

2 Remove all the pith from the grapefruit and divide it into segments. Chop and trim the segments and remove any pips. Retain the juice that comes out of the fruit as you prepare it. Fluff up the rice with a fork and stir in the prepared grapefruit and its juice. Add all the remaining salad ingredients and mix well. Keep on one side to serve with the trout when it is cooked.

3 Slash the trout across each side twice with a sharp knife. Brush inside and out with olive oil and season with pepper. Put the sprigs of mint in the cavity. Place under a hot grill and cook for 8–10 minutes on each side until the fish is cooked through.

garden paella

This recipe can be made with the vegetables alone but, if you like, you could add a small quantity of cooked chicken, shellfish or marinated tofu at the end of cooking.

2 shallots or 1 small onion, peeled and finely chopped

2 cloves garlic, peeled and chopped

1 teaspoon extra-virgin olive oil

1 very ripe beef tomato, skinned, seeded and chopped

¼ teaspoon powdered saffron

a pinch of cayenne pepper

175g (6oz) risotto or long-grain rice

8 bulbous spring onions

8–10 baby sweetcorn

400ml (14fl oz) good vegetable stock

75g (3oz) green beans

6–8 baby courgettes or patty pan squashes

75g (3oz) sugar snap peas

6–8 cherry tomatoes

1 Gently cook the shallots or onion and garlic in the olive oil until they begin to soften. Next, add the chopped tomato and cook quickly until all the liquid has evaporated.

2 Add the saffron, cayenne pepper and rice to the tomato mixture and stir well so that all the rice is coated.

3 Place the spring onions and baby sweetcorn on top of the rice and pour on the stock. Cook over a low heat for 10 minutes.

4 Add the beans, courgettes or squashes and sugar snap peas and cook for 10 more minutes.

5 Finally, add the cherry tomatoes and heat through for about 5 minutes. Serve from the pan.

duck slivers with orange beansprouts and chinese egg noodles

This is another 'East meets West' dish — a Chinese treatment of the Western combination of duck and orange. The very best duck to use is wild duck or mallard, as these birds have very little fat. Failing that, use a large Barbary duck breast and remove all the fatty skin.

1 onion, peeled and sliced

2 cloves garlic, peeled and chopped

0.5cm (¼in) thick slice of fresh root ginger, peeled and cut into thin sticks

1 teaspoon extra-virgin olive oil

about 2 tablespoons soy sauce

2 mallard breasts or 1 barbary duck breast, skinned and cut into strips

juice and zest of ½ orange

1 small red pepper, seeded and cut into strips

100g (3½oz) mangetout

a pinch of five-spice powder

150g (5½oz) mung bean sprouts

Chinese egg noodles (to serve 2)

1 Steam–fry the onion, garlic and ginger in the olive oil and a little soy sauce. Add the duck slivers and continue to steam–fry for about 5 minutes until the duck is cooked through. Remove from the pan and keep warm.

2 Cut the orange zest into very thin slivers and steam–fry with the red pepper and a little more soy sauce. Add the mangetout, orange juice and five-spice powder and cook for a further minute or so. Add the beansprouts and toss well together. Mix in the reserved duck and any juices.

3 Meanwhile, cook the egg noodles as directed on the pack and then serve straight away with the duck.

roasted red peppers with goat's cheese and sweet potato mash

Red is the predominant colour in this great match of flavours so I usually add a flash of green in the form of a chopped parsley and rocket salad.

2 large red peppers, halved and seeded

1 large clove of garlic, peeled and thinly sliced

2 tomatoes, halved

freshly ground black pepper (to taste)

4–5cm (1½–2in) thick piece Chèvre log, approx. 200g (7oz), cut into 4 slices

a pinch of dried thyme

SWEET POTATO MASH

2 medium to large sweet potatoes, approximately 400–500g (14–16oz)

2 level tablespoons Greek yoghurt

freshly ground black pepper (to taste)

1 Set the oven to 200°C/400°F/Gas 6.

2 Place the red pepper halves in a heatproof dish open side down. Bake in the oven for half an hour.

3 Turn the peppers over, put a few slivers of garlic in the base of each one and fill with half a tomato. Sprinkle with black pepper and return to the oven for a further 15 minutes.

4 Top each pepper half with a slice of goat's cheese and sprinkle with the dried thyme. Bake for another 5–8 minutes until the cheese just begins to run.

5 For the Sweet Potato Mash, place the potatoes in the oven with the peppers and bake for about an hour until they are cooked through. Split open the skins and scoop out the flesh. Mix with the Greek yoghurt and black pepper and serve with the Roasted Red Peppers.

Thai baked fish with steam-fried vegetables

This is a great way to cook almost any kind of fish.

2 fish steaks or fillets
1 large clove garlic, peeled and thinly sliced
1 stick lemongrass, cut into two or three pieces
1 red chilli, seeded and thinly sliced
juice and grated zest of 1 lime
1cm (½in) fresh root ginger, grated
1 tablespoon sesame oil
1 tablespoon soy sauce

STEAM-FRIED VEGETABLES
1 stick celery, sliced
½ green pepper, seeded and sliced
8–10 baby sweetcorn
50ml (2fl oz) vegetable stock
1 leek, trimmed and sliced
100g (3½ oz) mangetout
1 tablespoon soy sauce
50g (2oz) beansprouts
a few sprigs of fresh coriander

1 Wash the fish and place in an ovenproof dish. Arrange the garlic, lemongrass and chilli over the top of the fish. Mix all the other ingredients in a cup and pour over the fish. If possible, leave the fish to marinate for an hour. However, this is not essential.

2 Preheat the oven to 190°C/375°F/Gas 5. Cover the fish with foil and bake for 15–30 minutes, depending on the thickness of the fish.

3 For the Steam-fried Vegetables, steam-fry the celery, pepper and sweetcorn in half the stock. After a few minutes, add the leek and mangetout and the rest of the stock. Continue cooking until the vegetables are cooked the way you like them. Finally, add the soy sauce and beansprouts. Toss well and serve with the fish. Garnish with the sprigs of fresh coriander.

pot-roasted guinea fowl with spicy potatoes and wild mushrooms in sesame sauce

This is a good dish for a celebration. Guinea fowl has a more interesting flavour than chicken and it takes well to this simple method of roasting with all its own juices.

The wild mushrooms add a touch of luxury to the meal but if you don't want to spend quite so much you can use small closed-cap mushrooms with about 15g (½oz) dried porcini, or wild mushrooms, soaked in a little boiling water, to pep up the flavour.

1 lean guinea fowl, with as much fat as possible removed

2 tablespoons white wine

2 tablespoons vegetable stock

freshly ground black pepper (to taste)

a few sprigs of watercress

SPICY POTATOES

4 large baking potatoes

2 tablespoons extra-virgin olive oil

freshly ground black pepper (to taste)

a few drops of Tabasco sauce

WILD MUSHROOMS IN SESAME SAUCE

2 tablespoons tahini paste

50ml (2fl oz) soya milk

freshly ground black pepper (to taste)

2 large or 4 small shallots, peeled and chopped

1½ tablespoons extra-virgin olive oil

250g (9oz) wild mushrooms (e.g. chanterelles, girolles, ceps and trompettes des morts)

1 tablespoon lemon juice

3–4 tablespoons vegetable stock

some chopped fresh parsley

1 Set the oven to 200°C/400°F/Gas 6.

2 Place the guinea fowl in a heavy casserole and pour on the wine and stock. Add the black pepper and cover with a lid. Place in the oven and roast for an hour until the juices run clear when the guinea fowl is prodded with a fork.

3 Carve the guinea fowl and serve garnished with watercress. Pour the juices from the casserole into a gravy boat to serve as a sauce.

4 The Spicy Potatoes are roasted at the same time and same temperature as the Guinea Fowl.

5 Cut the potatoes into 2.5cm (1in) cubes with their skins on. Toss in the olive oil with the pepper and Tabasco and place in a roasting tin. Roast for about an hour, turning the potatoes once or twice.

6 To make the Wild Mushrooms in Sesame Sauce, start by mixing the tahini paste with the soya milk and black pepper in a small saucepan. Place over a low heat and slowly bring to the boil, stirring regularly. The mixture will gradually thicken. Do not cook for too long or the sauce will be too thick.

7 Meanwhile, cook the shallots in the oil for 1–2 minutes and add the mushrooms, lemon juice and stock. Cook for a further minute or two, turning the mushrooms occasionally.

8 Now add the tahini sauce, toss well together, sprinkle with chopped parsley and serve with the Pot-roasted Guinea Fowl.

jacket baked potatoes with tofu topping

A baked potato is a great base for a satisfying meal. Choose general-purpose or floury varieties such as Marfona, Maris Piper or King Edward, or try sweet potatoes for a change. All potatoes need to be well scrubbed and slit along one side with a sharp knife. Remove any nasty-looking eyes or holes.

You can bake potatoes in a microwave oven but I much prefer them baked in a conventional oven. This is because I like to have really crisp skins and this is impossible to achieve in the microwave. Of course, it is probably healthier to cut the cooking time and eat the potatoes when they are cooked but still firm inside! The choice is yours.

TOFU TOPPING

200g (7oz) silken tofu

3–4 tablespoons soya milk

1 tablespoon cold-pressed mixed seed oil

juice of ½ lemon

4–5 large springs mixed fresh herbs (e.g. basil, parsley and oregano or mixed parsley and mint)

freshly ground black pepper (to taste)

1 Place all the Tofu Topping ingredients in a blender and process until smooth and creamy.

2 Spoon generously over your cooked potatoes. Serve at once.

red mullet baked in a paper case

This is one of the ways in which red mullet is cooked in the South of France and you really cannot add too much garlic! If you prefer fresh herbs, use at least double the quantities (maybe a little more). Serve some boiled potatoes on the side.

a little extra-virgin olive oil

2–3 shallots, peeled and finely sliced

2–6 red mullet (depending on size), cleaned

3–4 tomatoes, skinned, seeded and chopped

2–3 cloves garlic, peeled and crushed

¼ teaspoon fennel seeds, crushed in a mortar

¼ teaspoon dried thyme

a pinch of dried rosemary

freshly ground black pepper (to taste)

2 tablespoons freshly chopped parsley

1 Preheat the oven to 180°C/350°F/Gas 4 and prepare two large double squares of baking parchment. Lightly brush the top layers with olive oil.

2 Place the shallots in the cavities of the fish and place half the fish on each square of prepared parchment. Mix all the remaining ingredients together, except the parsley, and spoon over the fish.

3 Carefully close up each parcel, folding the edges over so that no steam can escape. Place on a baking tray and bake for 20–25 minutes for small fish and 25–30 minutes for larger fish. Serve in the paper cases so that each person can unwrap their own portion.

4 Put the chopped parsley in a separate dish for each person to sprinkle over their fish as they unwrap it.

chickpea crumble with leafy avocado salad

Flavour and texture are all-important in this easily prepared, highly nutritious, main-course dish.

1 small onion, peeled and chopped

1 stick celery, chopped

½ small red pepper, chopped

2 carrots, peeled and chopped

1 teaspoon extra-virgin olive oil

a little vegetable stock or water

1 × 200g (7oz) can tomatoes

175g (6oz) canned chickpeas, drained

a pinch of ground cumin

CRUMBLE

100g (3½oz) wholemeal flour or brown rice flour

25g (1oz) oat flakes

1 tablespoon pumpkin seeds

3 tablespoons cold-pressed seed oil

LEAFY AVOCADO SALAD

mixed salad leaves

1 small or ½ large avocado, peeled, pitted and chopped

DRESSING

3 dessertspoons cold-pressed mixed seed oil

1 dessertspoon cider vinegar

1 Set the oven to 190°C/375°F/Gas 5. Steam-fry the onion, celery, red pepper and carrots in the olive oil with a little stock or water for about 5 minutes until the carrots begin to soften. Add the tomatoes, chickpeas and cumin and bring to the boil. Cover and simmer for 10–15 minutes.

2 Meanwhile, mix the dry Crumble ingredients in a bowl and rub in the seed oil until the mixture resembles breadcrumbs.

3 Pour the chickpea mixture into an overproof dish about 15cm (6in) in diameter and sprinkle the Crumble over the top. Place in the oven and bake for 30 minutes.

4 For the Leafy Avocado Salad, place the salad leaves in two small bowls and top with the chopped avocado. Mix the Dressing ingredients in a cup and sprinkle over the salads. Serve with the Chickpea Crumble.

potato, coriander and courgette pie

This mildly spiced dish needs a well-flavoured cheese for the best effect.

2½–3 tablespoons chopped fresh coriander
150g (5½ oz) Spenwood or Pecorino ewe's milk cheese, grated
1 clove garlic, peeled and finely chopped
1cm (½in) fresh root ginger, peeled and finely chopped
350g (12 oz) potatoes, peeled and thinly sliced
175g (6 oz) courgettes, thinly sliced
1 large onion, peeled and thinly sliced
75ml (3fl oz) white wine or vegetable stock

1 Set the oven to 190°C/375°F/Gas 5.
2 Mix the coriander, cheese, garlic and ginger in a bowl.
3 Line a dish with half the potatoes and cover with half the courgettes and then half the sliced onion. Next, spoon on half the cheese mixture. Continue with second layers of potato, courgette and onion, using up all that remain. Pour on the wine or stock and cover with foil.
4 Bake in the oven for an hour until a skewer finds the potato tender. Top with the remaining cheese mixture and finish off under the grill.

vegetable parcels with chilli sauce and kiwi salsa

It is worth making the effort to have a go at these attractive little parcels when you are entertaining. The quantities given here make 12 parcels or enough for four people.

75g (3oz) green or brown whole lentils
350ml (11fl oz) vegetable stock
75g (3oz) quinoa
175g (6oz) carrots, peeled and chopped
1 medium onion, peeled and chopped
2–3 sticks celery, sliced
125g (4½ oz) canned or cooked sweetcorn kernels
15g (½ oz) fresh coriander
15g (½ oz) fresh parsley
freshly ground black pepper (to taste)
24 squares filo pastry, approximately 20–22cm (8–9in square)
extra-virgin olive oil

CHILLI SAUCE
4 large ripe tomatoes, peeled, or 1 × 200g (7oz) can tomatoes
2 cloves garlic, peeled and crushed
2 fresh red chillies, seeded and finely chopped
a pinch of dried thyme

KIWI SALSA
2 kiwi fruit, peeled and diced
1 tomato, diced
1 small fresh red chilli, seeded and finely chopped
4 spring onions, trimmed and finely chopped
a pinch of ground cumin
juice of ½ lemon

1 Place the lentils and stock in a saucepan. Cover and cook for 10 minutes. Add the quinoa and return to the boil. Cover and cook for a further 15–20 minutes until the lentils and quinoa are cooked and all the liquid has evaporated.

2 Meanwhile, place the chopped and sliced vegetables in a steamer for 5 minutes over boiling water to soften them. Chop again and place in a large mixing bowl. Stir in the sweetcorn, herbs and pepper and finally the cooked lentils and quinoa. Mix well together.

3 Set the oven to 200°C/400°F/Gas 6.

4 Brush the squares of filo pastry with oil and arrange in piles of three. Place a heaped tablespoon of the vegetable mixture on each one, gather up into a money bag parcel and secure with a length of cotton. Place on a baking tray and bake for 15–20 minutes until well browned. (Remove the cotton before serving.)

5 Chop the tomatoes very finely and place in a saucepan with all the remaining sauce ingredients. Bring to the boil and cook over a medium heat, stirring from time to time, until the mixture thickens. Serve with the Vegetable Parcels.

6 Place all the Kiwi Salsa ingredients in a bowl and mix well. Leave to stand until required.

What You Need

Shopping List

Below is a general list of many of the bare essentials, standard necessities and other suggestions to put on your shopping list before and during your 6 Weeks to Superhealth. Most items are widely available in supermarkets, while a few are usually found only in healthfood shops. Choose organic ingredients whenever possible.

You'll have to look at the menu plans for each week and choose which meals you are going to have in order to do the particular shopping for those. The suggestions below are general guidelines and items that I suggest feature regularly in your shopping basket.

From Your Usual Supermarket or Shop

- Plenty of fresh fruit and vegetables – go for lots of greens plus a variety of colours, textures and tastes
- Fresh herbs e.g. parsley, basil, coriander, and spices such as ginger
- Mineral water (unless you have a filter or purifier)
- Oat flakes/porridge oats
- Natural, live (bio), organic, low-fat yoghurt
- Oat/wheatgerm
- Pumpkin, sunflower, sesame seeds
- Hazelnuts, almonds and other nuts (not roasted or salted)
- Lentils and beans, as well as other vegetarian sources of protein such as tofu products
- Brown rice
- Rye bread
- Extra-virgin olive oil
- Soy sauce or tamari

From a Healthfood Shop

- Quinoa
- Flax (linseed) and hemp seeds
- Buckwheat (soba) noodles
- Cat's claw tea
- Cold-pressed, unrefined sunflower/pumpkin/flax oil

Supplemental Options

To get started on 6 Weeks to Superhealth you will need:

Multi-vitamin and mineral – 2 per day for 6 weeks

Vitamin C – 1–2 per day for 6 weeks

Antioxidant – 2 per day for 3 weeks

Chromium – 1 per day for 1 week (optional thereafter)

Memory/mood support – 2 per day for 1 week (optional thereafter)

Cold pressed oil blend – 1 tablespoon a day for 1 week (optional thereafter)

The following companies all produce supplements of good quality. The products in bold on the chart (see page 214) best fit the recommendations.

Standard sizes for supplements are 30, 60 and 120s, so they won't always fit the duration of the programme. It's fine to carry on taking the supplement, even after it is no longer recommended in the programme, until the pot is finished.

The companies may offer a 'package' of supplements to meet all your needs for 6 Weeks to Superhealth. Please inquire with the company of your choice.

Higher Nature produce an extensive range of vitamin, mineral and herbal supplements that are available by mail order and may be found in some health-food stores. They also supply *Get up & Go* and *Essential Balance*. For mail order or a copy of their free catalogue, please contact: Higher Nature, Burwash Common, East Sussex TN19 7BR. Tel. 01435 882 880

Solgar produce a wide range of supplements available from any good healthfood store and some chemists. For stockists contact: Solgar Vitamins, Aldbury, Tring, Herts HP23 5PT. Tel. 01442 890 355

BioCare provide a wide range of good-quality supplements that may be ordered by mail. They are also available in some healthfood stores. For mail order or a free catalogue please contact: BioCare Ltd, Lakeside, 180 Lifford Lane, Kings Norton, Birmingham B30 3NU. Tel. 0121 433 3727

Health Plus produce an extensive range of supplements available by mail order. They also supply *Get Up & Go*. For further information and a free catalogue please contact: Health Plus, 30 Lushington Road, Eastbourne, East Sussex BN21 4LL. Tel. 01323 737 374

Seven Seas Ltd produce Extra High Strength Cod Liver Oil, rich in Omega 3 fats, available in chemists and/or healthfood shops. For stockists please contact: Seven Seas, Headon Road, Marfleet, Hull HU9 5NJ. Tel. 01482 375 234.

SUPPLEMENTS

	Multi-Vitamin/ Mineral	Vitamin C	Antioxidant	Chromium	'Smart Nutrients'	Digestive Enzymes	Cold-pressed Oil Blend
Higher Nature	*Advanced Optimum Nutrition Formula	*Immune C	*AGE Antioxidant Protection	*Chromium Polynicotinate	*Advanced Brain Food	*Easigest	*Essential Balance
Solgar	*VM –75	*Vit C 1,000mg with rosehips	*Antioxidant Nutrients tablets	*Chromium Polynicotinate	Phosphatidyl Serine	*Vegan Digestive Enzymes	
BioCare	*One-A-Day Multi-Vitamin & Mineral	*Vit C 1,000mg	NutriGuard Forte	*Liquid Chromium Polynicotinate	*Phosphatidyl Serine	*Digestaid	
Health Plus	*VV Pack	*Super C 1,000mg		*Chromium Picolinate		*Digest Plus	
Savant Distribution							*Udo's Choice

OPTIONAL EXTRAS

	Detox Formulae	Probiotics	Colon-cleansing Formula	'Female' Formula	'Male' Formula	Immune Complex	Omega 3 Fatty Acids
Higher Nature	*Terry's Herbal Aloe Detox *MSM	*Acidobifidus	*Colofibre *Herbal Clear	*Menophase *Pre-Mens Prevention	*Yang Drive *Prostaflorum	*Immune C	Omega 3 Fish Oil
Solgar	*Milk Thistle	*Multi-Billion Dophilus with FOS		*Herbal Female Complex	*Saw Palmetto Berry Extract	*Cat's Claw, Echinacea and Goldenseal Complex	Super EPA
BioCare	*HEP194 *HepaGuard Forte	*Bio-Acidophilus	*Colon Care	*Phytosterol Complex	*Prostate Complex	*Echinacea Complex	Mega EPA
Health Plus	*Milk Thistle		Absorb Plus		*Prostate Formula	*Echinacea *Cat's Claw	EPA
Seven Seas							Extra High Strength Cod Liver Oil

All products with * are derived from non-animal sources and do not use gelatin capsules.

Support and Resources

The Arica Institute

The Arica Institute, founded by Oscar Ichazo, offers one-day training in the exercise system *Psychocalisthenics*, plus other training. In the UK contact, Metafitness, Squires Hill House, Tilford, Surrey GU10 2AD, Tel. 01252 782661. In the US, contact the Arica Institute Inc., 145 Palisade Streeet, Suite 401, Dobbs Ferry, New York 10522–1617, Tel. (914) 674 4091 *or* Fax (914) 674 4093.

Essential Oil Blends

Essential Oil Blends containing a combination of cold-pressed seed oils are becoming more widely available. The best two products are Udo's Choice, distributed by Savant Distribution, 15 Iveson Approach, Leeds, West Yorks LS16 6LJ, Tel. 0113 2301993, and Essential Balance, distributed by Higher Nature who produce a wide range of supplements. They also supply *Get Up & Go*. Send for a free colour catalogue and newsletter to Higher Nature, Burwash Common, East Sussex TN19 7LX, Tel. 01435 882880.

The Institute for Optimum Nutrition

The Institute for Optimum Nutrition offers personal consultations with qualified nutrition consultants for those wanting tailor-made diets to help with specific conditions. It runs courses, including the one-day Optimum Nutrition Workshop, the Homestudy Course and the three-year Nutrition Consultants' Diploma Course. It also has a Directory of Nutrition Consultants (£2) which will help you to find a nutrition consultant in your area. For a free information pack, write to: ION, Blades Court, Deodar Road, London SW15 2NU. Tel. 020 8877 9993. Fax 020 8877 9980.

Natural Progesterone Information Service

NPIS provides women and their doctors with details on how to obtain natural progesterone information packs for the general public and health practitioners, and books, tapes and videos relating to natural hormone health. For an information pack, please write with stamped, addressed envelope to NPIS, PO Box 24, Buxton SK17 9FB.

Nutrition Consultation

For a personal referral by Patrick Holford to a clinical nutritionist in your area, please write to Holford & Associates, 34 Wadham Road, London SW15 2LR. Enclose your name, address, telephone number and brief details of your health issue. Alternatively, visit his website at: www.patrickholford.com

Meditation

There are a number of different approaches and courses available. Two that have received good feedback are the one-day Learn to Meditate course offered by Siddha Yoga Meditation Centre, 32 Cubitt Street, London WC1X 0LR, Tel. 020 7278 0035, and the courses offered by the London Buddhist Centre at 51 Roman Road, London E2 0HU, Tel. 020 8981 1225. Both groups have regional networks.

Supplement Companies

For a list of supplement companies and supplements that best fit the recommendations in this book, please go to Supplemental Options, page 213.

Psychocalisthenics

There are three ways to learn the entire *Psychocalisthenics* routine, other than following the indications in this book. These are, in order of preference:

Psychocalisthenics Group Trainings This is the fastest, most effective and enjoyable way of learning the exercises within a single day. The group energy facilitates this process and individual attention is included. For details of trainings in the UK contact MetaFitness (address below).

Psychocalisthenics Individual Trainings Expert instructors are also available to give one-to-one tuition. If you have a group of people who wish to learn *Psychocalisthenics* you can, again, arrange a teaching day with an expert instructor.

Self Tuition Kit You can teach yourself by ordering the self-tuition kit: the book *Master Level Exercise, Psychocalisthenics* by Oscar Ichazo, a video, a wall chart and a music cassette with voice guide, cost £58, available from P/CALS UK.

Master Level Exercise Video Part 1 provides instruction on each of the exercises. Part 2 is a run-through of the entire sequence with instructors leading a small group of people, making it possible for you to practise *Psychocalisthenics* using the video, cost £21.50, available from P/CALS UK.

For products, please contact P/CALS UK, PO Box 388, Wembley HA9 9GP, Tel. 020 8728 0211. Fax 020 8930 7311. E-mail: info@pcals-uk.com Website: www.pcals.com

For details on training or instructors please contact: MetaFitness, Squire's Hill House, Tilford, Surrey GU10 2AD, Tel. 01252 782661. Website: www.pcals.com.

MetaFitness also teach Chua Ka massage and can give you details of trainings and practitioners.

For overseas requests for products and/or trainings, please contact: Sequoia Press Inc, 250 Greene Street, Mill Valley, CA 94941, USA, Tel. (415) 383 6097. Fax (415) 383 6252. Website: www.pcals.com

For details on other teachers who give classes in other locations outside the UK contact: Arica Institute, 145 Palisade Street, Suite 401, Dobbs Ferry, NY 10522, USA. Tel. (914) 674 4091. Fax (914) 674 4093. E-mail: info@arica.org

Recommended Reading

You may wish to look into a particular subject in detail or get a more detailed overview of optimum nutrition, in which case I recommend that you read any of the following of my books, all published by Piatkus unless stated otherwise.

Optimum Nutrition Bible
100% Health
Beat Stress and Fatigue
Say No To Cancer
Say No To Heart Disease
Say No To Arthritis
Improve Your Digestion
Balancing Hormones Naturally (with Kate Neil)
Boost Your Immune System (with Jennifer Meek)
Supplements for Superhealth
The Optimum Nutrition Cookbook (with Judy Ridgway)
Mental Health and Illness – The Nutrition Connection (ION Press)

Index

Please note that any page numbers in italics refer to diagrams.

Ever wish you were better informed?

100% HEALTH NEWSLETTER & TAPE

If you want to be in the front line of what's new and exciting in health and nutrition there is no better way than subscribing to **100% Health**, Patrick Holford's newsletter. Considered the hottest voice in alternative healthcare today, Patrick Holford will share with you the very latest discoveries in a way that you can incorporate into your life. More of a journey of discovery than a journal, with each issue of his newsletter you'll have a new piece of the jigsaw of **100% Health**.

FREE-TRIAL NO-RISK SUBSCRIPTION Join NOW and receive a FREE newsletter. Your first issue comes free and, if you decide to continue your subscription, your subscription starts with the second issue. You pay £10 plus p & p a year and receive 4 newsletters. If you decide the first issue of the **100% Health Newsletter** is not for you you'll receive a full refund within 10 days of notification. Call +44 (0)20 8871 2949 giving your address and credit card details or subscribe by visiting *www.patrickholford.com*.

100% HEALTH SEMINARS

Take the first step to health by enrolling in one of Patrick Holford's seminars and workshops. These range from evening events to one day workshops on a wide range of subjects and four day intensives for doctors and other healthcare professionals. For a full schedule of events visit *www.patrickholford.com* or call +44 (0)20 8871 2949 for a list of events near you.

100% HEALTH CONSULTATIONS

For a personal referral by Patrick Holford to a clinical nutritionist in your area specialising in your area of health concern, please write to Holford & Associates, 34 Wadham Road, London SW15 2LR. Enclose your name, address, telephone number and brief details of your health issue. Postal and telephone consultations are available for those overseas. Full details are given on *www.patrickholford.com*.

See what others say about Patrick Holford's work:

'If you want informative, alternative information you can trust, Patrick Holford is the man. His work is completely brilliant.'   *Hazel Courteney, Sunday Times*

'Patrick Holford is guiding the nutrition revolution, Great work.'
                                    Dr Jeffrey Bland, Health-Comm Clinical Research Centre

'I am dazzled by the breadth of his nutritional knowledge. Patrick Holford has absorbed a tremendous mass of disconnected data and put it together in a simple way that makes immediate sense for the rest of us. Areas of complexity and confusion in nutrition are explained in clear, concise terms, understandable by all.'
    Dr John Lee MD, author of 'What Your Doctor Didn't Tell You About the Menopause'

'This is do-it-yourself health at its best.'   *Here's Health magazine*